Acclaim for *The Singing Bird*

D111123

"I read **The Singing Bird Will C** ......uue for the gift which Dr. John R. Noonan left to us. This book provides a rare, inside view of the experience of a sensitive and faithful man undergoing this increasingly familiar way of the cross."
—*Robert Ellsberg, Editor in Chief, Orbis Books*

"While this is a true account of a gay man with AIDS, I think it is a story that should be read by straight persons who have little understanding of gays or AIDS. It is easy for straights to dismiss gays as they do so easily. This account gives us an understanding that is badly needed in today's world. I learned much from reading this journal and hope others do, too. The basic lesson is: 'Judge not, and you will not be judged.' May Dick Noonan rest in peace."
—*Rev. Theodore M. Hesburgh, CSC, President Emeritus University of Notre Dame*

"This remarkable book by the late Dr. John Richard Noonan is a journal of discovery that probes the reality of his living with AIDS and of scanning the advent of death. His journal reflects the anguish, courage, self-honesty and faith with which Dick Noonan continued, despite the intensity of his suffering, to love and to sustain others, to celebrate life. He writes at one point: 'There is just no question—God is on the side of life.' **The Singing Bird Will Come: An AIDS Journal** affirms that all-encompassing insight."
—*Most Rev. Howard J. Hubbard, Roman Catholic Bishop of Albany*

"This is a book about accepting the reality of death each day yet living life to the fullest. It puts into words the journey of all those living with AIDS. Through his journal, Dick Noonan manages to open the inner chambers of his heart to provide a clearer understanding of what it is like to live with AIDS. He shares his experiences, so that all may share in and more fully appreciate the glory of the Paschal mystery."
— *Dr. Jane E. Dwyer, Founder and Director of Buddy Network Copresider of New Hampshire Ecumenical AIDS Taskforce*

"**The Singing Bird Will Come** is a very powerful journal. I am impressed with Dr. Noonan's gratitude for life and his graced acceptance of the blessings and tragedy it brought to him. The book is a strong testament to the power of family and faith."

—*Frank J. Cunningham, Publisher, Ave Maria Press*

"**The Singing Bird Will Come** is a welcome addition to the growing body of what might be called the testimonial literature of the dying. The memoir offers both heartache and comfort. Though Dick Noonan keeps a level head through the crisis of his impending death, the treasure of the book is in the well-balanced tension between dailiness and eternity. Who of us doesn't hope to catch hold of the splendor of the evanescent as we long for the consolation of the eternal? We look to the human connection to be reminded of our need for both and, even in death, Dick Noonan provides this connection."

—*Gregory Maguire, Author,* **Missing Sisters, Seven Spiders Spinning**

"This journal is the firsthand account of one man's struggle against a virus that ultimately ended his life. His words allow us an intimate glimpse into his relationships with family and friends, and how these relationships were changed by this life-threatening disease called AIDS. This journal is highly recommended reading for anyone: volunteers, case managers and other service providers involved with HIV/AIDS."

— *Anne Narciso, Director of Consumer Services*
  AIDS Council of Northeastern New York

"**The Singing Bird Will Come** is a story of courage and valor. It is a compelling account of an individual coming to grips with life, love, family and mortality. It will sooth the weary brow of all those living with HIV and AIDS and will be a blanket of warm memories for all those who love and care for them. It does the most important thing necessary and often overlooked in the world of HIV and AIDS—it provides hope."

—*Paul J. Donovan,* **Open Hearts**

The Singing Bird Will Come

An AIDS Journal

The Singing Bird Will Come

An AIDS Journal

by **John Richard Noonan, Ph.D.**
edited by **Mary Rose Noonan, CSJ**

with a foreword by
Daniel Berrigan, SJ

Canticle Press, Inc.
Latham, New York

Published by Canticle Press, Inc.
385 Watervliet-Shaker Road
Latham, New York 12110

⸺⚬⸺

⸺⚬⸺

Foreword by Daniel Berrigan, SJ
Cover Design © by Marion C. Honors, CSJ
Interior Illustrations © by Michael J. Noonan

⸺⚬⸺

Library of Congress Cataloging-in-Publication Data

Noonan, John Richard, 1957-1994.
 The singing bird will come: an AIDS journal/by John
Richard Noonan; edited by Mary Rose Noonan; with a
foreword by Daniel Berrigan
  p. cm.
 ISBN 0-9641725-4-2 (pbk./perfect)
 1. Noonan, John Richard, 1957-1994—Health 2. AIDS
(Disease)—Patients—United States—Biography. I. Noonan,
Mary Rose, 1951- . II. Berrigan, Daniel. III. Title
RC607.A26N65 1997
362.1'969792'0092—dc21
[B]   96-54910
                                                 CIP

Printed and bound in the United States of America
Second Edition

To our beloved mother
Kathryn Dwyer Noonan
who enabled the singing bird to come

~∞~

To Eddie, Rosemary, Ellen, Tom, Katy and Charlie
Edward, Jessica, Thomas, Michael, Brian
Emma Rose, Maxim, Elizabeth and Mary Rose
for the comfort of family love

~∞~

To Bob and Kevin
for the magic of childhood friendship

~∞~

To Gary, Barb, Jim, Maggie, Mike, John and Raymond
for the beauty of sustaining relationships

Acknowledgements

I am deeply indebted to many individuals for the publication of this work:

To my mother, Kathryn, my brother, Ed and my sisters, Ellen and Katy, whose love, courage and humor have been a source of life and inspiration to me

To my proofreader and friend, Sister Frances Patricia Degnan, whose skill, precision and commitment have been more the work of a coeditor

To our friend, Sister Patricia Houlihan, who enlivened Dick's hope for fulfillment in the promise of freedom to come

To my friends who read Dick's manuscript from many perspectives and gave me encouragement: Kay Smollin, Marla Yudin, Monsignor H. Charles Sewall, Sisters Katherine Arseneau, Charleen Bloom, Eleanor Ceccucci, Patricia Conron, Frances Eustace, Shawn Flynn, Karen Gaube, Joan Geannelis, Joan Teresa Groth, Katherine Hanley, Mary Agnes Kehoe, Mary Seraphine Meaney, Mary Theresa Murphy, Mary O'Brien, Roberta O'Rourke, Ellen Secci, Anne Bryan Smollin, Ellen James Spellman, Serena Thompson, Marguerite Tierney and Elizabeth Varley

To those who honored us through writing words of introduction and endorsement:
Rev. Daniel Berrigan, SJ, Mr. Frank J. Cunningham, Rev. Rodney J. DeMartini, SM, Mr. Paul Donovan, Dr. Jane E. Dwyer, Mr. Robert Ellsberg, Rev. Theodore M. Hesburgh, CSC, Most Rev. Howard J. Hubbard, Mr. Gregory Maguire, Ms. Anne Narciso

To Marion C. Honors, CSJ, and my nephew, Michael J. Noonan, who enhanced the work through their artistic talent

Finally, to the Sisters of St. Joseph of Carondelet, Albany Province, whose support made this publication a reality.

The writing of Dick's journal was the work of one man. The publication has been the work of many persons who shared their suggestions with and confidence in me from the start. Thank you so very much.

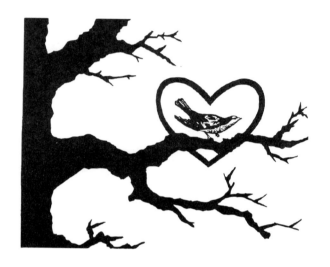

If I keep a green bough in my heart,
the singing bird will come.
—Chinese proverb

Foreword

We have here a testament of the love that overcomes—in this instance overcomes the harsh, omnivorous empery of death.

Death, as someone has said, is not *something that happens to you*; it is *something you do.*

I like that. It casts light on the death of Christ, the deaths of our death-ridden century as well. Death is something you do. In an important sense, the statement de-demonizes death, mocks its inflations even, brings it down to size, makes it *manageable,* a task to be done.

To be done well, as in the lives of the martyrs and saints. Death was a task Romero did well, and the murdered nuns of Salvador, and the Jesuits. A task which in our country, Cesar Chavez and Dorothy Day and Thomas Merton did. And so well!

Between these covers is a testament to a task done, and well done.

Knowing that he was dying, face to face with death for a long time, increasingly weakened and ill and dependent, a young man overcomes.

He overcomes the terror that death, that great necrophiliac, commonly summons, with its hallucinations: a rattling of chains, a showcase skeleton leering, an hourglass and scythe in hand, and claiming like the ghost of an irate sheriff: *Pay up!*

Death, dying rather, is a double task to be done (in reality, one task). First, a hardy spirit must set itself to exorcising the above awful images.

As a preliminary. If such images are to be evicted, there are infinitely better ones, straight from the imagination of Christ, to replace them.

Welcome to the banquet of the Realm—*My Body given for you; My Blood poured out for you*. Welcome to the harvest of good Wheat, to the Bridegroom at the door, to the Pearl in hand, the Treasure uncovered in a field.

The man who wrote these pages died well. The proof is in the reading: the serenity and hope, at times, the sheer laborious overcoming. A Himalayan climb—but then the glory!

How grateful we are, that such a spirit as his, for awhile, shone brightly, lived among us.

Lives among us, rather.

Daniel Berrigan, SJ
New York, New York

Preface

For our brother, John Richard Noonan, the knowing began on September 28, 1989. On that day, he joined the then 100,000 Americans in whom the AIDS virus was ticking away.

When sorrow and pain brought Dick to confront his humanity, he dug into the core of his being and was propelled toward life. He reached inward to discover a remarkable strength that enabled him to view his task of dying, in all its challenging and frightening moments, with striking clarity.

In his journal, Dick describes simply and directly his reaction to living and dying with AIDS: his physical deterioration and mental anguish, his successes and failures in connecting with family and friends, his moments of grace and his times of near despair, and the emotional and spiritual suffering that accompanied his search for peace.

To its very end, Dick's writing reflects a psychologist's insights into the private and public events of the AIDS world. He reports advances in medical research and notes afflicted famous figures. He articulates his ardent wish to beat the odds, yet recognizes the common fate he shares with so many other individuals. He cautions himself against bitterness but faces the reality of harsh, anti-gay sentiments in the general population.

Like most stories of the human condition, Dick's is one of joy and heartache, laughter and tears, victory and defeat, pain and hope. It is a journey of an individual's striving for wholeness even as his body falls apart. It is a journey from head to heart, a journey toward freedom to be one's true self and, most of all, it is a journey Dick did not anticipate so soon.

—MRN

September 20, 1989

Yesterday was my thirty-second birthday. The day started with a call from Mary Rose, continued with a good day at work, and concluded with calls from Mom, Mike and Katy. I called Ellen because I had forgotten completely that her birthday had been the day before mine. By the time Gary came home from work, it was too late for us to prepare the dinner he had planned—lobster tails and filet—but we did have a cake and presents: a sweet Hall sugar bowl and a coffee grinder. It was a wonderful birthday.

Today Gary's HIV-test results came back positive. (He had gone to the doctor with some diffuse, fluish symptoms.) He called me in the morning to tell me he had found used tires for the truck, and that his results had come in (a bizarre combination of news); he couldn't see the doctor until 4:00 p.m. I asked him to call me regardless of the outcome. Today is Wednesday, my long day at the clinic. My mind raced all day, and by 5:00 p.m., when I had an hour free, I was jumping out of my skin. When Gary hadn't called by then, I knew. Still, I had a welcome walk from work to the restaurant. It was a beautiful evening. The leaves are falling here now, and I passed a houseful of sorority kids singing awful songs to an assembled group in their front yard. In spite of myself, I was surprised that my heart was at peace. I actually believed that things were as they were supposed to be. There was a lot of sweetness in that walk. My world still felt like a gentle place.

When I arrived at the restaurant, Gary said, "I don't have good news." I said simply, "I know," and went on to an appointment while he finished his day's work. Later on at home, we watched television while I picked out photos for the videotape M.R. is making for Mom. I pulled out pictures of me as a baby and as a little boy, posed with Dad and Eddie, Mom, Gram, everybody. All these people love me, but right then, I felt very unlike the person in the photos, the one they love. In the last two years, I have come to terms with myself and my life; yet I haven't shared those feelings with the people I love. There are no pictures of that. My own test results will come back in two weeks, maybe sooner. I expect them to be positive—if not this time, then the time after that or the time after that. It's so hard to tell my family. I'm afraid they will think my life is hard, sad, ugly. Even now, with Gary's testing positive and my not knowing my own health status, even now, I can't persuade myself that I am a sad case.

I'm writing my journal as a sort of fantasy that someday I might give it to someone, and you may know the *me* I didn't have the nerve to tell you about. I'm sorry for that. In reality, however, I probably won't give these thoughts to anyone. Writing just helps sometimes. A while back, I realized that I felt as though my whole life were an adventure into which I had been launched with no idea of the outcome—not exactly an original thought but what **was** new for me was my excitement about it. Now I know a little bit more, though still not much, and I'm afraid sometimes. I repeat the Serenity Prayer *ad nauseam*, adding "Thy will be done," and I'm surprised each time to realize that this prayer expresses exactly what's happening to my spirit.

September 21, 1989

These days seem so long. Today I am writing in the evening. Gary is working a double shift. In a little while, I am going to the restaurant *Comedy Night.* Not much seems really funny, but we'll see.

I find most things very tiring these days. As soon as I get a second free, my mind swings back to AIDS and everything I don't know yet. I'm so afraid of what will happen to us. We just arrived in Canton and don't really know anyone here. We came here to build our lives together, not to end them. I think of how and where to bury Gary and how hard it would be for him to die here in the North Country. Right now, I'd like to return to North Carolina where at least we have friends. The worst thing I can picture today is Gary's dying first and my eventually returning to Utica to wither away in front of Mom and everyone else.

Of course, none of this is relevant today or needs deciding. I know my choices will be clear when they will need to be so, but right now I am fighting that "It's-not-fair" attitude. I think every young child learns that life is not fair and almost as early understands sadly that equality and justice are not really primary in the natural scheme of things. My body is reteaching me both lessons every day.

September 22, 1989

I dressed this morning and found myself staring at Gary's body as he slept—his leg sticking out from under the sheet in its usual way, his sweet, handsome face—and the feelings of love for him that always surprise me came to the surface. It is a real amazement at how much I want to know his heart more and more. Mom used to talk about a kind of wonder she felt upon seeing us as babies—how she was awestruck by the look and smell and perfection of our bodies and the incredible development of our minds and spirits. Though the feelings aren't exactly the same, the similarity I see must have something to do with my being a gay male because I never felt this way with a woman. Maybe I simply have never been truly in love before, although I thought I had been. The strength of my emotions overwhelms me, and I'm grateful, really, for a depth of feeling I didn't remember I could experience. At the same time, I feel suddenly and blindly furious that somewhere beneath that beautiful frame, something is at work trying to kill Gary. So what did I do? I kissed his forehead and gave him some coffee, and he took me to work. It's wonderful when feelings of love and warmth peek out at the beginning of an ordinary day.

September 25, 1989

We just finished a great weekend. I bought a nice carpet remnant on Saturday to lay on the stairway and in the hall. Yesterday Gary had the day off; we hit an auction and bought a table lamp, ironing board and electric frying pan. In the afternoon, we stopped by the restaurant and bought two wicker armchairs, two loveseats and two tables—not sure I'm crazy about the wicker, but at $15 a piece, it's admittedly a cheap way to furnish the place.

We had a good talk on Friday night—made plans. When Gary gets really sick, he doesn't want to be here in Potsdam. I agree. We came here to build a life, not to end one. We will probably return to North Carolina, so that Gary can be closer to his sisters and where the support of friends we don't have here yet will be a help. From the look of things, if I am infected, I'll probably outlast Gary. I can either stay in North Carolina or go back to Utica. It amazes me that I sit here writing this stuff. In a couple of weekends, we will be celebrating our first anniversary—barely at the beginning of our time together, and we are planning the end of it. There is something strangely embarrassing about this for me, as though we're teenagers posing as a mature couple; instead we're healthy young men acting like an old couple. Is dying together made more meaningful by the length of time you live together? I think not. This disease is going to rob us of our middle ground, the time when my family and some of my friends might have looked at us and said, "Yes, they are a happy, faithful couple, and their commitment lasted." More than anything right now, this is a disease of bad timing; I know that's an understatement.

Gary has decided to contact a specialist in Syracuse to see what should be done about the swollen lymph nodes in his groin. The acute pain in his leg and the sweats that started this whole thing three weeks ago are not a problem now, though he does say he can still feel the pain in his leg, and the lymph node has changed in size.

One of the things that amazes me most about our newly found knowledge is that I wonder whether or not I will ever have another day when AIDS and our life together aren't the major issues of the day. Though I feel that we have done a remarkable job of coping in a short time (and I really do), behind every move—buying a carpet, going to work, reading a book, watching a movie—is the thought, "Should I be doing this? Gary could be sicker at any moment." I miss the recent past when I didn't worry about absorbing meaning from every moment of life.

September 26, 1989

Often I am surprised to get what I ask for in prayer. This probably happens more often than I know since I either forget to pay attention or actually forget what I prayed for! Anyway, yesterday went by, and I barely thought of this whole situation; when I did think of it, it was with a calmness unusual to me. In fact, I talked with Mike last night and broke the news to him. A first! Someone else knows about Gary now. From the beginning, Mike and I were able to talk well and freely. I didn't snivel, and he didn't panic, although I know the topic scares him more than he can articulate. Actually, I find that my major concern in telling others is how the news will hit *them*; that's an answer to my prayer—not to forget others as we deal with our own end. I am going to have to learn to trust that others will deal with the pain this news causes them in the best way they are able.

Anyway, Mike told me about Hurricane Hugo which did a lot of damage to his parents' place in Charlotte, and I talked about Gary and me. My life has been touched over and over by many good and gentle persons. The rest of the day was good and mundane; I went through an unproductive day at the clinic, picked up the house and gold-leafed a lamp I had bought at the auction this weekend—a day of bliss bereft of import. I'm learning how much more I need to rely on God and trust more in the coping strengths of my family and friends. Maybe soon I will be able to talk more freely about my life.

September 27, 1989

It's a beautiful fall morning. There was frost on the windshield for the first time this year. The air, the sky, the colors of the trees all seem a little sharper than usual. You would have to be dead not to notice the beauty. We're not.

Gary called from work last night to see whether or not I wanted to go to the movies. A man we had recently met came into the restaurant and invited us. We went to see *Sea of Love* which I hated. Pacino was never one of my favorites, and seeing Ellen Barkin, whom I normally find fascinating, didn't do a thing for me. Her cold, slanty mouth, usually quite sexy, looks in this movie as if she has had a stroke. The reviews seem to like the characters but found the story, especially the cheap ending, rather implausible. I didn't care for any of it.

Since I was just about to eat something when Gary called, I had nothing for supper except popcorn. When Gary pointed out that I hadn't been eating well, I suddenly became irritated about everything, looking for someone to blame. I can feel myself wanting to get angry but needing a reason that won't make me sound foolish. I caught on to what I was doing before I actually did or said anything and gave myself over to Gary's sweet efforts to make me feel better. It worked, thank God. Sometimes it seems as if I am always sad or angry or worried these days. Occasionally, though, it starts to occur to me that I don't have to take care of everything. God really *does* take care of my life; so what's the big deal? I'm grateful for those moments. Right now, my life is quite good.

It is Wednesday night, and as I wait for my last client to come, I know I am lonely. It is getting cold out, and this time of year always reminds me of coming home from school or from my friend's house to our own warm home. I want to go back there tonight. I want to sit with my mother and have her hug me. I want to tell her how much I love her. I want her to know that her love has been the one constant in my life. But tonight I can't call anyone with this news and my sadness; someday soon, I will have to make those calls. During times like these, I feel as if my life has been designed to hurt the people I love the most. I love you, dear Mother, and you, Eddie, M.R., Ellen, Katy. I'm so sorry for any pain I cause.

September 28, 1989

A beautiful morning! I feel good for no particular reason and don't question that feeling. On the drive to work, Gary and I talked easily about living and dying. It didn't seem monstrous today, didn't feel as if we were hapless victims of a cruel God. It felt calm and real and OK. I still believe it has been a good, gentle world for me (It took a lot of struggle to get to this belief.), and the major harm that can be done now is the harm I do to myself. Gary and I are *not* victims or tragic heroes. We're a couple of guys who still have a place in the world and are working to appreciate that place as best we can. I am blessed. I hope I will remember that.

September 29, 1989

Yesterday I got the results of my test; I am HIV-positive too. Gary cried. I didn't cry until later when Gary was at work; actually I think this news hits in a place deeper than tears. I felt a profound sense of loneliness, wanting to tell my family and trying to figure out how and when to tell each one. Maybe it would be better to wait at least until I have symptoms.

I am sad for the things that won't happen. Our relationship won't be long enough now for my family to see that it was a good, enriching, faithful one for me. I'm afraid that people will limit their thinking to just a couple of guys who managed stupidly to kill each other. We are so much more. There is respect and happiness, goodness and love.

I think the poor lady at Planned Parenthood (where I had my test) has not had to counsel HIV-positive folks too often

(Thank God), and I wonder if she were scared. She asked what I would be doing after our meeting and was oddly surprised, I think, to hear I was going back to work. She counseled me to stay as immune as possible, to get as many vaccines as my doctor thought advisable, to get a TB test and to stay away from sick people. Later on last night, I actually started to laugh thinking about our conversation; it reminded me of the joke Gary and I had developed when we read in the almanac about the speed of the fatally poisonous black mamba snake versus that of a human being. It felt as if she had just told me there was a black mamba on my tail that could go 30 miles per hour and would be chasing me at least that long. Her advice: "I suggest you sprint."

I slept well last night, in spite of the news, and went to work as usual. Once in a while, I catch myself in surprise when I realize there is a virus cooking away inside me that will leave me dead. I am left to remember that I am as special as my mother always told me I was; I am so much more than a strong chorus of confederated cells. Unfortunately, however, the virus doesn't know this. I don't understand the scheme of things, don't even insist that there be one, though I believe there is. I want this not to happen to us, to anyone; I am **not** indifferent to it. I cherish my life and want every minute that's coming to me. I want to continue my life with Gary, to keep loving my family and friends, to watch my nieces and nephews grow up, to see another summer at the lake, another fall in Potsdam. I want all those things, but I know, too, there is so much more in the eternal scheme of things.

One other thing occurred to me today. I don't believe in dying; I believe in death. Dying isn't the complementary side of living or the opposite side of it. As best I can tell, it is exactly synonymous with living. My dying didn't start when they told me I was carrying HIV, and it won't end if they tell me there is a new cure for the virus; it began 32 years ago when I started living. Therefore, I dub this process *living* which I intend to keep up until and long after you can't see my breath on the mirror; so there is no real room for dying. I hope I remember that. Here's the final scene in the movie version of my life. The doctor emerges from my hospital room to address my huddled, weeping loved ones: "You had better hurry in. He's *living*."

I read this over and am surprised to find at least two examples of humor; I wonder if that's odd, especially since I **do** feel as if some of this is rather funny. I try to suspend the humor and get really angry. An insidious virus is challenging my right to be here! A quieter, much gentler voice from somewhere answers, "Relax. The virus is just a means; it isn't hostile; it has no energy; it doesn't care. Your right to be here is unchallenged. Your right to be here was never guaranteed. You know that." I *do* know that. I *do*. And I can live with it.

October 2, 1989

Today is the first anniversary of Gary's and my meeting. October has always been a kind month to me. It has been an amazing year. Gary and I had breakfast Saturday with Tom, a local guy who seems pretty solid. He asked how long we had been together, and I think was surprised to hear it had been only a year. To most persons who know us, it looks longer. In fact, it seems longer, too. Somewhere along the line, I committed myself to this guy. I guess I could get along without him, but I don't want to have to do that.

I was reminded of my feelings this weekend. Gary wasn't in a great mood, and I don't always understand his moody days— partly because they are so infrequent, and partly because he is not really accustomed to talking much when he is in them. In any event, I found, to my surprise, it didn't matter; I still wanted to be around him. Maggie always said I was like a creosote bush, that when I want to be alone, I spread a toxic cloud to guarantee it will happen. Gary doesn't do that.

The act of writing seems to force me into a kind of focus. I hope to pick and choose what is worth mentioning, though I can't say I remember to do that when I pick up the pen. What does seem true, however, is that I want not to waste space listing my gripes. It is easy to defend the idea that the world is full of insensitive, uncaring, selfish individuals. AIDS is not my enemy, nor is death. What is dangerous is my own tendency to nurse grudges in the belief that it is I who sees all things clearly.

I think I say all these things because I have just finished a book recommended to Gary by a local woman whose son died of AIDS at the end of 1986. She details the last two years of his life, describing the events they faced as he died. The disease is, of course, horrible, and I can never know the feelings of a mother who has lost a child, although I have counseled many. I am sympathetic to this woman, but I am struck by the bitterness and anger on every page of the book, emotions so strong that they even obscured my view of her son. It seemed to me her prime motivation for writing the book was to get some kind of revenge, to take the opportunity to name all the persons who didn't respond to her son's illness and death the way his mother felt they should. If "there is a time for everything under the heavens," maybe this book came into my life to show me how **not** to react. I have to hold on to the belief that love and life are stronger than bitterness and death.

I have prayed so much in the past few weeks for the same things over and over again: for Gary and me, that we may die with faith in ourselves and in what will come next, for my mother who I know has passed on to me everything I need to live and to die well, for Eddie, M.R., Ellen and Katy who love me beyond words, and for the grace to do God's will at every moment from now on. And today, if I have a specific prayer, it is that I don't become bitter, that I remember it is not how far short we fall that matters, but that we try in the first place.

Dear Mother, if the time ever comes that you're asked to see me die, no matter what I say then in my weakness, I am grateful to you and Dad for my life. Please know how much I love you, and stay at peace.

October 3, 1989

We might get wet snow tonight. I'm excited about the idea of winter this year. Given our situation, Gary and I talked over the weekend about how to approach the apartment. Actually, I like his attitude. I had toyed a bit with a "What's-the-point?" approach, reasoning that if we save money, we will be "more ready" for when we get seriously sick. Gary said rather simply, "This home may be the only one we'll ever have together. I'd like it to be nice." That puts it into perspective. Besides, we're not talking here about thousands of dollars.

We had an off-the-cuff anniversary dinner last night. I threw it together while Gary was still at work: nice breaded, seasoned pork chops, noodles Alfredo, salad, croissants and gingerbread with lemon whipped cream for dessert. Gary set the table, and it looked beautiful. Then we watched *Beaches* on the VCR—an OK movie except for its being too long and too unbelievable. What's going on with Barbara Hershey's lips anyhow?

October 4, 1989

I am booked straight through today at the clinic with no breaks; so the day should pass quickly. Last night I worked on finishing the new bed and catching up on the laundry. A while ago, I read Noel Coward's diary and couldn't figure out how he did all he did in a day: "wrote the score to *Pacific Overture* this morning; had lunch with Binky and Duff—charming as always; Marlene came for tea—she's being a silly bitch again; wrote *Hay Fever* all afternoon and went to the theater tonight." Well, back to the *Lifestyles of the Poor and Unsung.*

Kate's going to the hospital today to be treated for a suspected tubal pregnancy. She sounds good about it, but there is a lot of concern in her voice. I hope they don't have to take the tubes. Mom got in the car as soon as she heard and was there in Ithaca when I called. I feel stuck; I can't figure out when there will ever be a *good* time for my *bad* news. Eventually I might be forced by circumstances, but maybe I'll see an opening earlier than that. I know it seems unfair not to tell them. It's just that I have conducted my life separately for the past couple of years as far as being gay goes. Now they get to be around to pick up the pieces. The only trouble is: they weren't supposed to be among my broken pieces. Then I think of exactly how many of the tens of thousands of diagnosed cases of AIDS have been in exactly the same position and am struck by the sadness and confusion and pain which I (and soon, I'm afraid, my whole family) have in common with humanity. It's a strange comfort. Thank God, I'm not unique in this case.

October 9, 1989

It's back to work after a long weekend. On Friday, Gary and I drove to Syracuse for his appointment with the specialist. Gary felt really good about the visit and was impressed by the doctor, who had him see another specialist immediately, and who ruled out a femoral hernia on the swollen lymph gland and was glad Gary had not opted for a biopsy at that point. The plan is to let the swelling go down on its own. The doctors aren't sure whether or not the gland is a result of the virus but have decided that Gary is asymptomatic for AIDS at the present time. We'll go back in a month and then orchestrate treatment with a doctor up here.

Saturday I spent the whole day cleaning the apartment and forgot to eat something until 9:00 p.m.—too late to save me from some real grouchiness. I asserted to Gary in my best open-communication fashion that I was angry because he wasn't giving me enough help around the apartment. He basically ignored my anger and then told me he did a lot around the house. Right on both counts! Of course, there is no question in my mind that my anger is always justified (in the sense that I can justify it!), and just as true, that there are times when I itch for a fight.

Last night Tom and I went bowling. It was only he and I; the attendant found our lack of expertise riotous. We both edged over 100 in our two games, scores which Gary found hilarious when he heard. I'm glad to have gone out with Tom. I get lonely without friends here—we had so many in North Carolina—and must open myself up a little more.

At lunch time today I took a walk down by the river across from the clinic. It's the kind of day I was hoping for over the weekend: sky a brilliant blue, air the clear, light-sweater type. I sat and watched a gaggle of Canadian geese swim around. The fall leaves would soon drop into the water to be carried away quietly, gently, rightly, somewhere to a place we don't know. I felt a part of things.

Sometimes now I actually invite Death to sit next to me, and we have a conversation. Though I do, indeed, picture robes which obscure its face, Death isn't at all silent but has a voice which responds to my questions:

"Why do you do it?"

"It's my job. I have a place in the order of things, and I try to do it well."

"Why me? Why Gary? Why the persons I love?"

"Oh, please. No offense, but why not? You're a pretty nice guy, but you don't expect the leaves to stay on the trees because of that, do you?"

"You seem rather unfair sometimes."

"In truth, I think so, too. Sometimes I feel good about what I do; other times, I don't understand it myself. Remember, I'm just a conduit, a vehicle. I'm not God, you know. I'm just Death."

"So why am I talking with you?"

"Good question. You started it."

"What are you like under the hood?"

"The truth? I'm lonely. I'm viewed in many ways: proud, cowardly, powerful, scary, mysterious, cruel. And what I really am is lonely. The living understand me even less than I understand myself; the dead pass by and are gone. They stay with me long enough for a quick touch, not even an embrace, as living poets claim."

"So why do you keep the job? You sound as if you hate it."

"Nobody else can do it so well as I. I'm uniquely suited to it. There are benefits, too."

"This conversation is getting too cute. The benefits?"

"Well, yeah. Like travel."

"Ok. A Barbara Walters question: If you could be a tree, what kind of a tree would you be?"

"Anything but a weeping willow."

"Any advice for me?"

"Yeah. Don't talk to me too much. A little is OK. You don't know much about me because you're not supposed to know much about me. Learn to get comfortable with, maybe even to celebrate, what you don't know. And don't worry too much about getting ready for us to meet again. I'm never early, and I'm never late. Being prepared is just your way of exerting a control you don't have. Give it up and enjoy living instead."

October 11, 1989

More and more, I write for comfort. I got home last night, and Gary had soaped "I love you" on the bathroom mirror. One of the best parts about the love I have for this man and my knowledge of its reciprocity is that it puts me in mind of other faces, other times when I knew about love. Somewhere along the line, I had forgotten these moments and what they signaled. For a short time, I cried easily and then got a bit hard. I can't put an exact time on when this all began, but it was around the time I left for Notre Dame. So many things happened that year. Mary Rose entered the convent; Dad died; Eddie and Rosemary got engaged; Ellen and Tom met at St. Rose. Anyway, Mom and Katy took me to the Syracuse airport; I started crying when I kissed Mom *good-bye* and couldn't stop for a long time in the air. It had been a year of just the three of us since Dad died, and I didn't want to go away. Then something happened, and I could feel myself drawing away somewhat but not knowing the reason. Since that time, all I have ever done is hold the gap from widening at the same rate it began. Now I know the reason, and I'm a different man, but I just haven't shared much of that person with those I love most deeply.

I love you, Mother. I remember your putting notes in my lunch bag that said those same words. I remember crying often at the thought of being different from all of you but not knowing exactly how. Please know that my efforts to live my life honestly and with integrity result from the love all of you have shown me. Thank you for giving me your own glimpse of faith that says clearly to me now, "There is much more to come."

October 13, 1989

Friday the thirteenth. Last night I had a good time running the assertiveness group with Barb. The preceding day, we had worked together on a couple's case. Afterward, she told me she really admired my work. Funny, it seems so long since I had heard that from anyone. The compliment buoyed me up for the next two days. Noticing that other persons do things well and commenting on their skill shouldn't be so difficult as it is—judging by how infrequently we compliment one another. I, too, need to do better with this form of connecting with other persons.

After group, Gary asked Tom over for dinner, and we tried our hand at bowling again, something I had never done with Gary. Although he hadn't bowled in years, he obviously had been good once. I am extremely competitive and hate showing off my inexperience. Still, when I let myself be teachable, I actually pick up useful tips. I hope I remember that when I am dying. Why would I be good at bowling? I've done it maybe four times in my whole life. And why would I be good at dying? I've never done it. One can always hope.

October 17, 1989

Tuesday afternoon. After an amazing day yesterday, filled with hot winds that stripped most of the trees, today is very cold and wet. And tomorrow, forecasters are predicting snow—three seasons in three days. Move to the Northeast to escape boredom! Already, today seems designed to search out, corner and destroy my good mood.

Sunday night, Gary and I watched the HBO special *Common Threads: Stories from the AIDS Quilt*. I had started to watch it while he was at work but couldn't stand to watch it alone; so I stopped the VCR until Gary got home. I'm still finding my way through the mess of feelings I have. It sounds odd to me, but I was so grateful to see the two men whose lovers had died and who both now have AIDS (One has already died and was clearly very sick when they shot the film.). I keep assuming that Gary is farther along in the disease than I am and will be the one to get sick and die first, and I am scared. I can't picture my life then. I don't want to drag my sorry self home to Utica to die amidst my heartbroken family, although I know what many persons in the same boat don't know—that I would be welcome and loved. Many persons never have the chance to think of all these things. I'm not sure which ones are the lucky ones.

We were struck by the strength of the individuals interviewed and the remarkable beauty they found in life. There is hope for us.

Also, I found myself panicking over the lack of evidence, after we die, that we had ever been inhabitants on the earth. If the producers of the AIDS quilt were to come to our house after

Gary dies, what would I show them? I want to guard his memory, prove he existed and was important to someone, and I want him to do the same if I should die first. Eddie and Ellen and Katy are leaving a living legacy in their children; M.R. is giving the best of herself to the community she loves. What will I do? I want to write but don't know exactly what to say. I want to rent a camcorder but don't know exactly what to record. And I want to hurry it all because what if one of us starts to get that AIDS death look soon? It is as though I want to record every step of a monstrous climb because I'm afraid I won't recognize the descent. I know this is an odd way to view life because I really think there are no ascents, peaks or descents that matter much anyway. In the end, there is simply the realization that love, wherever one finds it, is a treasure worth telling about. And maybe I **will** become, through my family's memories, a parent of a different sort. Maybe, through stories of me, my life **will** bear fruit for generations to come.

Yesterday I took a day off because spending time with Gary had suddenly taken on a new importance. It was warm and windy, and we took a walk around town in the afternoon. I felt very much the hooky player and loved every minute of it. By 3:30 p.m., though, Gary had to get ready to go to work, and I let my mood slide. First I started thinking I had wasted the day and had accomplished nothing of value. Then I threw myself into frenzy of cleanup which made my mood worse but the house much better. By the time Gary arrived home, I was grouchy and looking once more for a reason to bite his head off. Happily, I refused to let myself find one.

October 18, 1989

It is 5:30 p.m. on my long Wednesday, and I am tired. I finish at 7:00 p.m., just after my next appointment. This day went by quickly, mostly, I think, because when I arrived at my office, I really wanted to work. God knows, I have enough paperwork to keep me busy, and it has done so.

We had our first major snowfall last night. First, I think of how much I had missed the snow up north when we lived in North Carolina; then I think of how much I miss my friends down south now that we live in Potsdam. It's not an equal trade-off. Tonight I don't want new friends; I want my old friends. I want to go home but am not sure where home is. The self-poverty with which so many of my clients struggle every day hits me hard.

When we arrived home from work, we heard that San Francisco had suffered a major earthquake just as we were being belted with the snow. It is very tempting to look around and see the world as a harsh place; confirming the impression with my own self-pity, I know better. Even as I write, I know there is sweetness and gentleness and care out there for me. I will try to pay better attention.

October 19, 1989

Payday! I have looked over the budget for this paycheck, and it is amazing how far we have come since we moved here. It is heartening also to see what a team we have become. Maybe "team" isn't a good word because there is no unhealthful competition. We shop together, decide about the house together and agree on where to go financially. We may not get there, but who cares? Gary says it is the most secure he has felt in years and, surprisingly, I have the same feeling. I suppose I could do this by myself but, thank God, I don't have to do that. Gary has brought so much into my life. I think I've never articulated my idea of a good partnership before this time, but somehow I've tripped across it anyway. No, that's not strictly true. We have worked hard on this relationship. It may be even more than we are due, but then who decides who is due what and when? I do know that today I am overwhelmed with the gift of my life, and if something as stupid as a paycheck sparked these feelings, that's fine. I am frequently stupid and should be so more often; there is definitely a new sense of urgency in my life.

October 22, 1989

It's Monday morning after a good weekend. I spoke with Mary Rose on Friday, and I think she and Mother are coming up in a few weeks. I think I can pull the place together by then. Most of the major work has been done.

Gary is now general manager at the restaurant. He feels proud and scared at the same time; he has worked hard this past year, and it is heartwarming to have that effort recognized. We sat down and talked money on Saturday. I have budgeted us through 1990. By the end of next year, we should have saved a considerable amount of money, something neither of us has experienced in a long time. We may end up doing the bed-and-breakfast thing after all. It doesn't hurt to dream.

The doctor called Gary on Friday to say he is not sick (by laboratory standards) at this time. Gary was relieved to say the least. His T-4 count is 570; so low-dosage AZT (Azidothymidine) is recommended at levels from 300-500. Supposed normal range is 500-700 or so, Gary tells me. I guess there is no telling, or at least he wasn't told, when one with a 570 count might reasonably expect to drop below 500. We go for another visit in a few months. In the meantime, I feel fine.

I told sweet Maggie about our situation this weekend. That means she and Mike are now the only persons who know. Maggie cried and wanted us to come "home" to North Carolina. I wound up crying, too. Though we are building our life here at least for the foreseeable future (Whoever coined that expression probably got hit with a meteor two minutes later.), I was so happy to hear someone say, "Come home." I know my mother will say the same thing, but still, during a period when I feel as though telling my family would hurt them more than it would help me, that phone call made my life immeasurably better. Thank you, Maggie. I love you and am grateful for you. I hope there is peace for you in this life.

Sometimes I get the urge in these pages to talk about my memories as though writing about the present has sparked a new interest in my past. Maybe I will; maybe I won't. Suffice for now to say here that I have more flashes of happy images than I had ever realized, and they help me immensely now. If I think of my life as a song, some of the lyrics are banal, uninspired, ordinary, even hurtful, but more often I am struck by the beauty of some of the words and music. In any case, today I'm still humming, and that's enough right now.

October 27, 1989

An incredibly beautiful Friday for this late in October! Beautiful skies and about 70 degrees! In fact, all week has been Indian summer. I hope it holds out through the weekend. On Sunday, we're going down to Syracuse to see *Les Misérables,* and I can't wait! Then we'll get ready for M.R. and Mom's visit next weekend. I think they will like the apartment.

Last night, we went to hear a man who is HIV-positive talk at Potsdam. It was very strange for me. One would think I would feel a common bond with this man, but I didn't. Maybe I have to feel sick first, or maybe I wouldn't have anything in common with him anyway, and the fact that we have the same virus doesn't join us in spirit either. I suppose our humanity should join us, but that's not the feeling I walked out with tonight.

My strongest feelings right now about being HIV-positive are quiet and private. They are precious to me, and I want to share them but only with some persons. The quilt stories on TV felt like that to me, too, and I was amazed at those individuals' abilities to show pain or anger or happiness quietly and without declaring themselves pained or angry or happy. I don't know exactly what I mean here. I want not to be anyone's lesson in anything simply because I have the virus. I wouldn't mind being a lesson because of my life, but the possibility or likelihood of that seems rather slim, given the number of persons who know that much about me; besides I have no idea myself what my life's lesson teaches others or what I would have it teach them. I do know, however, that the virus doesn't qualify me to sit on a stage and be the object of pity, scorn or even admiration. It's a virus, not a medal.

I don't know exactly why the speaker bothered me. Partly, it is my own discomfort with displays of emotion at that public a level. I felt like a voyeur; he felt to me like an exhibitionist. It seems the audience thought him special, maybe even a little creepy, the same attraction that brings high ratings to Geraldo, Donahue, Sally Jessy Raphael, etc. I wonder if people think *good actor, great director* and *great photographer* when someone mentions Rock Hudson, Michael Bennett or Robert Mapplethorpe. They become *the actor, director and photographer who died of AIDS.* I want my life defined in terms other than those of my sickness and death. If someone remembers me at all, I would wish it to be in terms of the happiness, the faith, the love I gleaned just from the opportunity to be here for a little while. I don't feel tragic, and I think I'm not.

November 2, 1989

I haven't written in nearly a week. This hiatus has less to do with nothing happening than with too much happening.

We went to Syracuse this past weekend to see *Les Misérables.* It was wonderfully staged, and the performance was terrific. The seats, excruciating in their lack of leg room, were the major problem at the theater. Still it was a great trip. We have had good times in Syracuse tucked into the medical visits.

I have had time to think about myself, not in a selfish way but in an evaluative way, in a way to predict how I might face my future. I know I'm still becoming, though at times, I can't wait to see what. In a good sense, however, I have already become a person of whom I am proud. I am the kind of man who actually intrigues me. There are times when it seems I know very little about myself; at other times I know a lot more. Certainly, there will be much more to know in the next few years.

Mom and Mary Rose come the day after tomorrow. The frenzy of preparation is almost over. I hope they like what they see.

November 20, 1989

It's been two and a half weeks since I have written. For the most part, I think this is a good sign since I hope it means I am less obsessed with AIDS. At the same time, I need to write precisely because if it is true my life isn't about AIDS, then there should be other things about which to write.

There are, of course. Mom and M.R.'s visit was a wonderful time. I think they really liked the place, and they were such fun company. By the time they arrived, I had given up on major improvements and had settled for the much-needed hanging prints, hanging plants, buying new sheets and so forth. We had a great time looking at the furniture I had refinished. Gary had arranged reservations at the restaurant, and we had a delicious dinner. There is just no better company than my mother. I received a really sweet thank-you note from M.R., who, I think, is allowing me space to open up. I just want them all to see how happy our life is together before I break the news, and we both feel fine and look as good.

I have just finished reading *And the Band Played On*, the Shilts' book on the story of AIDS, its epidemiology and the response by this country: government, public health, medicine, gay factions, everyone. It's a long book, but I finished it in three days. I realized about halfway through the book that I was looking forward to an ending that I knew I wasn't going to find: that the virus had stopped spreading, a cure had been found—something that would deny my own personal reality. After reading the book, I experienced mixed emotions. It did some good to read and re-alize again that the virus is now so widespread that I am just taking my place in a long, sad line. Somewhat to my surprise, I find I *do* have feelings of shame, of punishment. The metaphor that Shilts kept using was that the early victims of AIDS, those with promiscuous backgrounds, were the early victims because they had been "dancing in the freeways." Sometimes, it is hard to remember that I didn't do that. The idea of punishment doesn't fit at all with my concept of a God of love and mercy and forgive-ness.

Tomorrow we go to Syracuse to see the specialist; I go for the first time, Gary, for the second. I find I want to write that the visit is not prompted by the spots which have suddenly shown up on Gary. I keep telling myself that these are not KS [Kaposi's Sarcoma] lesions, that they can't be and then start explaining to myself the reasons for which they can't be: They don't look like any KS I have ever seen. (Now I am a world-renowned cancer specialist.) There are too many, too fast (Though hardly reassur-ing, this actually seems true.). The spots look like a rash or an allergy. And my triumphant *coup de grâce*: they're not purple, and they are supposed to be purple.

I realize I am bargaining in a fairly obvious way because I feel unready to accept the fact that these lesions might actually be KS and the consequences such as "OK, OK, I've got it; we're both going to die of AIDS, probably Gary first, but not just yet, OK?" Let's face it, I have never in my life felt ready for the really scary stuff, even when I knew it was coming. Though I pray for courage, I believe it is not a subjective experience or feeling, such as, say, happiness or sadness. If there is a feeling connected with courage, it is probably fear; if there is a behavior, it is probably **not** doing what the fear tells you to do. So I am going to Syracuse tomorrow even though, or precisely **because** I am suddenly coming up with so many good and completely transparent reasons **not** to go.

November 22, 1989

Yesterday we went to Syracuse to see the doctor. Although he wasn't really expecting Gary for another few months, the doctor checked Gary's bumps and summarily dismissed them as infected follicles. Gary was relieved but is still poking and prodding himself every day in a sort of ritual combination of fear and precaution. On the whole, though, he is in good spirits. Last night, he asked me to feel a bone in his chest and to tell him if I thought it was a bone, if it was supposed to be there and why there wasn't one on the other side. I told him, "Yes, it is a bone; if it is there, we are going to assume it belongs there or has a very good reason for relocating, and who the hell knows why there isn't one on the other side." Then he said, "I think I'm becoming a hypochondriac." I said, "Of course, we both are, and it's probably a normal reaction under the circumstances."

My visit was fine. I like the doctor's manner—calm, laid back and friendly. In addition, he seems reasonably knowledgeable, and that has become more important to me now that I know there is more information out there for those who are motivated enough to look. One of the early casualties in myself (from which I am slowly recovering) is my belief in people's good will in the advance of AIDS research. I was struck to see *And the Band Played On* in the bargain bin at the Watertown Mall, a $35 hardcover selling for less than a Stephen King paperback. It had never occurred to me that there are individuals (some of them important) who might make a difference and who would happily let me die even though they don't even know me. I have always tried to teach my clients that one doesn't love other persons in spite of their imperfections but because of them; the warts make us human and join us in compassion and solidarity. I wonder if saints and angels enjoy one another's company? I hope so; it will be fun to get love and trust back endlessly.

When we met, the doctor asked me how I was. I replied, "Fine," and then he asked, "Really?" And yes, really, I am OK. I told him I was there just to make sure that I was as OK as I felt. After the exam, the chest x-ray, the EKG and the bloodwork, he gave me his AIDS, talk complete with options and game plans. Well, really, there is only one option, one game plan. When my T-4 count drops below 500, we go for AZT in low dosages—DDI maybe, if I can't handle AZT or if I have been on it a good while, and it starts to look as though it is not working. Is this the start of something?

November 24, 1989

Yesterday was Thanksgiving. Gary had to go in to work for only about an hour; so we had most of the day together. Tom came over after dinner at his mother's house. He is such a nice guy and the closest thing I have had to a friend (besides Gary) since I moved from North Carolina. I spoke with Ellen, and it looks as though Tom got the Kansas City job; he will start soon, and they will all move this summer. Mom called, and I talked with her, Eddie, M.R., Ed, Mike and Brian. We had a wonderful day, sweet and quiet. Gary picked the place up while I cooked, so that by dinner time, it looked as if the table were set for two really neat people. I did the works—turkey, cornbread stuffing, gravy (with giblets for me and without for Gary), broccoli soufflé, carrots and beans, mashed and sweet potatoes, baked bread and pumpkin and black-bottom pies. Afterward we just sat around and watched *It's a Wonderful Life* for the hundredth time, crying like fools. Then Katy called; so I had Thanksgiving conversations with all the persons for whom I am most grateful.

For whatever reasons, we are just in the right tempo of things and are now ready to start Christmas shopping. Even more amazing, I have already bought gifts for Ed, Mike, Thomas and M.R.

and know what I'm getting for Brian, Emma Rose and Jess. I'm going to arrange baskets for the adults and am going to make an appointment with the photographer today. I want to give everyone a photo while I still look good. My life is a gift. Today I realize that more than I have ever realized it before. I won't worry about tomorrow.

November 27, 1989

I seem to feel good these days when I write in my journal. Sometimes I wonder whether or not my timing is responsible since typically I pull out the notebook when I have a few extra minutes at work. Would it be different if I wrote at home? The miracle is that I feel good most of the time; so I think it would make little difference when I write. The fact is that I am in a state of emotional upheaval very seldom these days and, even more mercifully, the simple act of writing neither requires nor induces such a state. I can look at my life now, and I don't fall apart; in fact, I am still proud of what I see.

Thanksgiving gave me the chance to realize how loved both Gary and I are and how, without realizing it, we have touched and have been touched by more lives than I ordinarily stop to consider: my family, my friends in North Carolina and finally some new friends up here in the North Country.

I bought the Sunday *Times* and took it to the restaurant to read while I waited for Gary to set up the place. We went home and ordered a pizza to enjoy while we watched a crummy horror flick. This is a quiet, ordinary life we lead, and it is wonderful at the same time. I wish people could realize that our fidelity, just like that of any other couple, is forged out of the ordinary stuff of daily existence.

November 28, 1989

Scratch the good-mood-when-I write idea. I am looking out the windows at some very ominous skies, hoping somehow that the weather will rescue me from work today. This is far from impossible although it is unlikely. All I'm asking for is the predicted 50 mph winds with freezing rain!

Last night I went to the restaurant to wait for Gary, sat in one of the wicker chairs facing Main Street and listened to old music. Potsdam has a postcard of Market Street at this time of year. The Christmas lights are in the windows and the snow is falling, looking much like a movie set. The music was sort of sad, old pop-folk tunes like *Where Have All the Flowers Gone, Carolina on My Mind*—pieces virtually guaranteed to leave you mellow. A little voice in the back of my head kept saying (*Saying to whom?* I remember asking.), "But I **like** my life."

Today I overslept and rushed to work just in time for my first appointment and followed it with a two-hour intake. This is the first time I have sat quietly by myself, and I am so sad. I'm not so intent on exploring or explaining the feeling this time. Maybe I'll just let it take its course; it's not fatal. Sometimes I feel like one of those old European still-life oils where the flowers are next to the fruit which is next to the dead rabbits. I'm about contours and textures and nuance; some of my elements are jarring, even alarming. I try to remember it is the **whole** that is a thing of beauty, really quite exquisite. It's too bad that sometimes I have a lousy memory.

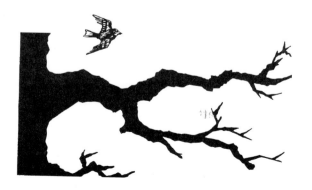

November 29, 1989

Lately I feel my denial of our infection rebuilding. There is a funny sort of balance I keep looking for but probably wouldn't recognize it if I found it. There hasn't been a day since September when thinking about AIDS hasn't occupied at least some of my time. That may never change, although in reality, I think it is taking up less and less time. It's just that now when I **do** think about it, I think either, "Maybe we won't get sick," or "Maybe it won't be fatal for us." I have started buying the *New York Times* because I figure the Syracuse paper might not carry potentially important news, and then I worry that the *Times* doesn't give a damn either. The papers have been full of long stories about how a few individuals have come down with a red-blood-cell sickness and how the public-health agencies have mobilized into quick action, identifying bad batches of L-tryptophan. Is the pursuit of help for this disease of mine on the right track? Would the response from the government and the research community have been faster and more integrated had the AIDS virus shown itself first in a day-care center or a little-league camp rather than in gay men? I think so. About all I know is that the reported cases in the United States are over 112,000, and that officials have discovered huge numbers of unreported cases. About the only information I get from the *Times* is contained in the obituaries. I'm very discouraged tonight.

December 12, 1989

Nearly two weeks have gone by since I've written. Christmas shopping and work have been taking up most of my time. Lately I seem to be stuck between desires to do good things for myself and a *What's-the-point?* attitude that follows closely on the heels of the healthful desire. So, even as I go through another spasm of self-disgust over my smoking, I use this infection to say, "Why bother stopping?" I use it, as well, to avoid getting back into working out, even though I am definitely feeling the effects of not having done it for three and a half months. Of course, the infection excuse is just a new variation of a very old theme. I prop up excuses as to the reasons I can't or don't do good things for myself; in that sense, it is like the ultimate self-destructive dream come true, if only because it is *almost* but not quite believable. I've never found the perfect excuse for squandering my days.

December 18, 1989

The last week before Christmas. I found out over the weekend that I threw a rod on the truck, and it needs a new engine. After the initial panic over the lamentable timing of the Fates or Furies or whoever it is who disables trucks, I realize that I've never been in a better position to deal with it. We had a wonderful weekend in spite of the truck. Yesterday we put up the tree, exhuming the lights from last year's Sad Café Christmas and getting out the balls. (I bought two boxes of irregulars for $1.00 at the end of last season!) I remember rummaging through those boxes finding the best balls I could and then buying a big roll of red ribbon to make bows for the branches. What a lovely reminder that things **do** get better! So the tree is up, the decorations are out, and tonight we'll buy the remaining presents. I think doing all these normal holiday preparations serves as needed evidence to me that Gary and I can go on as we did before we knew there was a virus ticking away in us.

December 25, 1989

Another Christmas has come and gone. All in all, this one was special for sure. For one thing, I actually bought and wrapped seventeen gifts in time for the holiday. Much better, though, was Gary's and my Christmas together. We exchanged presents Christmas morning and then drove to Utica; so now Gary has met every one in the family and has spent his first Christmas with us. I had a strange mixture of feelings while I was home at Mom's.

On the one hand, I was very excited to have Gary meet my entire family and to have them meet him. At the same time, however, I sat there realizing the essential dishonesty of our presentation to them diminished some of the joy for me. They don't know how much I love this man and how happy and grateful I am to have that love. I suppose this is just an elaborate way of describing a half-full glass from the wrong perspective. If everything I wanted wasn't there, most of it was. And my family picks up so much without my telling. They had gifts for Gary as well for me. I find myself wondering if a happy ending is possible. And what exactly *is* a happy ending?

January 8, 1990

Wow! The first entry of the nineties, and we are both healthy! I refinished, repainted and lacquered an antique table Mom had given me for Christmas and painted the Hoosier cabinet and chairs in the kitchen. Now I need to do the other three chairs, table and stand-up cabinet. The new year is bringing new hope.

The big news is I haven't had a cigarette in six days, and my sleep improved immediately; it is both more restful and more dreamfilled—quite nice. It is easier getting out of bed in the morning too. The other noticeable difference is an almost immediate circulatory improvement; my hands and feet are warmer. Maybe all these things point to a good year.

April 3, 1990

Today, when I think about the whole AIDS ordeal, I am simply struck by the work it will take to "get things in order." What a hilarious, absurd expression! I know what I mean by it: telling everyone at the right time (God knows what obscure invitation I will rely on to let me know when the right time is.), trying to figure out how to keep insurance in effect, wondering where to die, how to save people I love from pain (another bad joke of a notion, I know), etc. At times, my fantasy is just to get sick, cross the border into Canada, drive north until the population thins out and then sort of disappear like a diseased, old animal going away to die. Since it probably won't work out that way, I hope I'm OK with however it does work out.

What's equally on my mind today is Mike's upcoming visit, the possibility of Maggie's spending vacation time with us, my workshop in Rochester and our trip to Florida. It's all about connections and somehow not dropping stitches I have already knitted—far more interesting than obsessing about the yarn still in the ball!

I love our apartment. When the HIV tests results came in, I thought one of the big inequities was that we found out the bad news so soon after moving up north. I felt more "equipped" in North Carolina than I felt when we first arrived in Canton. I don't feel that way anymore. I look around and see that we are doing what we came here to do—build a good and happy life together. And I love that.

April 9, 1990

It's Monday morning, and morning is the hardest part of the day for me. Between the time I get up and the time I go to work, the disease is nearly all I think about. It's there when I shave, when I shower and when I dress. This seems to be true every day; it is as though I am required to do a certain amount of digesting of the whole picture before I can begin my day. What's worse these days (and maybe it's because I'm dulled by sleep, and my defenses are down) is that the thoughts seem to present themselves in new and particularly unpleasant ways.

This morning it occurred to me that if Mary Rose's condition worsens and Mom gets sick, in some not-too-far-off span of time, Eddie, Ellen and Katy will be attending three funerals and will be all that's left of what we thought was a fairly large family.

And I sometimes hate myself for being the unnecessary, avoidable death and for causing pain to those who love me and whose lives will go on.

This particularly unhealthful reflection comes, perhaps, as a result of talking with both Mother and M.R. yesterday. Reflexively, I talked about how good I was, and I feel as though I am giving them a tour of the foyer of my life. I don't know why I can't trust my family and my friends with the beauty of some of the other rooms, like the depth of my life with Gary, or allow them the pain of still other rooms, like my HIV status. I guess it's my house, and I have the right to do that; it's that old worrying about the timing again.

Ryan White died yesterday. Strange—I was listening to National Public Radio while I painted the front door, and when they did a brief editorial/memorial, I found myself saying aloud to him, "I wish you peace and freedom now." This disease provides the usual opportunities for individuals to behave like heroes, victims, jackals, whatever, I guess.

April 19, 1990

I went down to Pittsfield to see Ellen and Tom for Easter. It was a rather impulsive trip that I decided to take on Holy Saturday. I actually called hoping El might invite me down, which, of course, she did. I had a terrific time. We went out for Easter dinner and afterward took a walk around Stockbridge. Then, while Ellen packed treats for my trip back, Tom and I studied a map for the best return route. It was just a wonderfully ordinary family celebration complete with a wonderfully extraordinary niece and nephew, and it was just what I needed. I'm happier for the comings and goings in my life.

June 13, 1990

It has been almost two months since I last wrote—a time of vacation in Florida and entertaining out-of-town friends in

Potsdam. I'm writing as I wait for the last appointment of the day, having been in a fit of work since I returned from vacation. So far this week, in addition to paperwork at the clinic, I have refinished a library table, an oak chair and a telephone table. We decided to be optimistic and renew the lease on the house for another year; we did put on hold our thoughts of buying a house; I guess that's called tempering optimism with a touch of reality.

I read in the *Times* that the incidence of fatal PCP in AIDS cases is down; as persons with AIDS begin to live longer, they now die more frequently of Kaposi's and other causes. That's neither good news nor bad news; it's just news.

Gary and I continue to live out our lives in a tiny little part of the country where our situation, were it known, would still be a curiosity. The trip to Rochester last week made me wish for a bigger place where we could have friends who are like us. Still, more and more, I have come to feel at home here. I like going to work, and Gary is rightfully proud of the strides he has made. In many ways, I feel we have accomplished the purpose of our move, and I am grateful to the area and the people here for giving both of us that chance.

So, why am I lonely tonight and even a little sad? I think the reason is that I'm tired of the secret part of this. I'm tired of not knowing how things will go. There are too many emotions jockeying in my heart, especially the one that battles over whether to continue fighting or to let go. Is letting go the same as giving up?

I remind myself that my *today* is calm and sweet and good, but I'm still sorry that those feelings won't last much longer. I need to try to stay a gentler course.

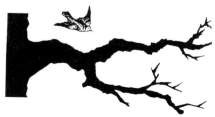

June 15, 1990

I was so tired today, and what a shock I had. When I got out of bed, I had a terrible, albeit brief chest pain when I took a breath. Everything nice disappeared. "Oh, my God, it's here. I have pneumonia." Well, it is 5:00 p.m. now; I'm still breathing, and I have had no pain since that first one.

Have I written in this journal how I find myself praying for intentions again? I stopped using intercessory prayer for a while because I had convinced myself that God doesn't quite work that way—by answering some prayers and ignoring others. I thought, "Thy will be done" is a much easier and much less disappointing prayer. Anyway, I'm back to asking God for a few things like "Save Gary and me from much pain," "Give me the grace I need," and "Bless my family with peace." I even thought of praying that Mom would die before I died because that seemed kinder and easier. Then I quickly decided that that prayer stemmed from my own chickenheartedness and was an insult to her own good faith. Lots of times, I just ask God to help me to keep my eyes open to the love and goodness in my life.

June 28, 1990

Mom and Mary Rose have asked me to serve on the medical advisory board of the newly formed Central New York Chapter of the United Scleroderma Foundation. I accepted, of course, because I would do anything to help M.R. cope with this disease, but I'm scared at the idea. They don't meet for the first time until next April. I found myself wanting to back out and explain that I don't know what I'll be doing next April. By then, they might find themselves organizing a Utica Chapter of the AIDS Foundation. I hate the fact that I'll have to hurt them sometime soon with my news. It makes me think that maybe some of the persons with AIDS have no family support because they disappear from the scene to make it easier on everybody. It's just nice to keep things as normal as possible for as long as possible.

July 10, 1990

We spent Wednesday through Saturday at the lake and celebrated Mother's birthday. The kids are growing up so fast. The picture I made for Mom was a big hit. We saw everyone but Katy, and I talked with her on the phone.

Yesterday we went to see the doctor in Syracuse. He told me that if my T-4 count were still in the 400s, I should start AZT. I was staggered because he hadn't gotten back to me after my last visit to tell me that the count was so low. At that time, I guess I still associated AZT with full-blown AIDS cases only, to which it is no longer limited. I wonder what the count will be when I get it next week since it was 446 the last time. If the AIDS virus reverses the T-cell ratio and measures an immune-system dysfunction, will it ever really climb back significantly? I think not.

The upshot of all this is that I'm coming closer to being sick. I knew enough before not to be seduced into thinking that I would be ready to hear bad news just because I had given it so much thought. I wasn't and I'm not. It was like getting mugged. You know they are going to kick you again, but that doesn't keep it from stunning and hurting you when it happens.

My news was upsetting to Gary who was very concerned and anxious. I figured he would be the one to get sick first. Sometimes, especially when I think about telling my family the bad news, I allow myself to think that, with all the surprises, it might just be possible that someone will come up with a lovely little drug that will stop this virus dead in its tracks and restore me to my forever immunological bloom. I no longer dwell on that thought, however; it is hard enough taking some of these developments in stride without specifying the kind of miracle for which I pray. I continue to think that I get my miracles in many different forms. It is only when I hang onto a specific one that I run the danger of bitterness and disappointment.

July 13, 1990

I spent the last two days home from work sick. I *think* I was sick anyhow. The correlation between my feeling ill and the doctor's news on Monday is a little hard to miss. It is difficult to tell whether I was more scared than sick or the other way around. It is harder still to tell whether or not that matters.

What upsets me is how much it bothers me to be sick. I keep thinking, "This is as good as you are ever going to feel. From here on in, it gets only worse." Wednesday night, I got to sleep only after a long time of praying for some peace and quiet in my life.

Ironically, Gary seems to be getting stronger. I guess that is ironic only if I am the center of the universe, and when I have a bad time, everyone else is supposed to have a bad time. What worries me is that right now I want not to hear about other people's sorrows or joys. I'm having a hard time getting pleased or excited about things that would give me great joy under normal conditions. Please God, I hope it doesn't turn out that I am a person who is that weak.

July 23, 1990

I don't know whether or not it is starting. The doctor called Friday, and the news wasn't good. My T-4 count is now down to 309; so the AZT is a go. I felt I was prepared to hear a number under 500, but 309 sounds awfully low to me.

I had told Barb midweek of my situation because I was tired of Gary's being the only one up here who knows. She was and continues to be a wonderful friend and made me promise I would talk to her when I needed to do that. Barb helped me in a special way by giving me the name of a local pharmacist who, she felt, would maintain confidentiality.

The AZT comes in tonight. It's a scary feeling. I can't believe that I am actually going to begin to take an AIDS drug. I can't decide if it is the nightmare or the reality of the situation that is shaking me up so badly. The doctor says my chances of getting pneumonia escalate considerably when my count goes below 200. I quickly calculated that, at this rate, it would be below 200 by Christmas—not a good mental exercise to have undertaken.

I got a call from Tim who wants to get together this fall in South Bend for a ND football game. I was noncommittal, being somewhat unsure of how to say, "Gee, Tim, I'd love to go if I'm not dying of AIDS by then." I enjoyed talking to him after such a long time but was angry with myself for being embarrassed, guilty and secretive to so many persons who, I know, would do their best to understand my situation.

So, what are my biggest complaints right now? With a count of 309, I don't have a lot of energy and am occasionally a bit lightheaded with lots of joint and muscle aches. If I didn't know what I know, I'm not sure I'd even notice any of those symptoms. Knowing what I *do,* however, I seem to scan myself a thousand times a day for symptoms. And I'm praying for courage and balance because I think I need both gifts badly. I try to take one day at a time to learn more fully what it means to be a human being, and I reflect on a piece of Dan Berrigan's poetry:

> *Each Day Writes*
> *in my heart's core*
> *ineradicably, what it is to be man.*

July 27, 1990

It's Day Three of AZT. The stuff sits on the bathroom shelf over the sink; so I won't forget to take it. I said to Gary, "This makes me feel like a little old man." I'm 32, but I go through the day now trying to remember when it is time to take a pill. Starting when I get up, I take pills every four hours until I go to bed. It's quite bizarre to look at a bottle of 150 pills and then read the label which says, "Five refills." I guess this is the long haul.

I was thinking the other day about the unlikelihood of my lasting this thing out. I couldn't think of too many good reasons for which I might survive when so many others haven't made it. I'm a nice guy, but there is nothing especially compelling about me that would call off the last days.

At the same time, however, I can, from my own life, make a strong case for the existence of grace, miracles and forgiveness. There have been everyday moments of tremendous joy and love and kindness, for all of which I could never have thought to ask; so those moments are the reasons my biggest prayer is usually for the ability simply to notice and pay attention to those big and little moments. While I can't persuade myself that maybe I'll get out of this because I'm such a great guy, I can allow the possibility of it based on the graces I've received already, without asking and, in many cases, undeserved.

July 30, 1990

The pain in my leg which started on the fourth of July and which I had hoped was a deep bruise, worsened over the weekend. For the first time, it bothered me even when I was lying down. I went to the doctor, and he wasn't concerned about the leg—said it would go away in a few days. He did report, however, that my liver enzymes are up, although nowhere near where they would be if I had hepatitis. We did discuss pneumocystic prophylaxis if my T-4 count drops below 200. Except for my leg, I really feel OK and have begun working out again.

I seriously thought of going to Ithaca to tell Katy about my situation and asking M.R. to be there, too. Then I decided against it at this time.

August 20, 1990

We went to Montreal this weekend where I attempted to satisfy Gary's curiosity about Catholicism. We visited Notre Dame Cathedral and St. Joseph's Oratory. Gary enjoyed the whole thing.

The cathedral is magnificent, of course, and he loved seeing the bishops' tombs. He was thrilled to see the cardinal actually doing a baptism and was only mildly disappointed that he wasn't wearing a red biretta. I was struck, quite unpreparedly, by the power of the place. I knelt and prayed and cried—not a sobbing mess but quietly. I was a bit embarrassed when a sweet-looking nun shot me a most wonderful, kind smile on the way out.

I didn't know what to pray for; so I just told God how confused I am by all this. I don't know whether or not I'm accepting it the right way, but I don't know how to do it any better either. I do know that on some days it is getting harder to accept my life as pure gift, and I feel unusually sad on those days. I'm trying to remember the important things, but it is often difficult to figure out what those are, too. They say that Goethe's last words were "More light." I'm not dying yet, but I surely could use a little more light.

At Brother André's tomb, I had a hard time separating show from substance, but Gary loved it all. It's a good place to vent a little anger at God who must have been watching as all these pathetic-looking individuals crawled up the many stairs with hopes of a miracle. I felt as if it were a lottery at which climbing the stairs on your knees gave you a better chance than the $1.50 votive candle, and the lucky winner throws down his crutches

It took a little while for me to regain my perspective. Recognizing the power of God in my life and the presence of grace has, indeed, made me freer and happier and more peaceful. I think I'm looking for tiny little miracles and a deeper, inner peace. And I hope the same now for these candlelighters, kneecrawlers and tombgrabbers. They and I are one.

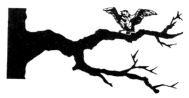

August 31, 1990

I made flight reservations to go to North Carolina where I'll stay at times with Mike and at others with Maggie. I have developed a weird habit of planning trips; so I'll have something to look forward to and then immediately hope I don't get sick in between with little bouts of pneumonia. Of course, these periods never end; there is always another bargain to strike. In addition, I have discovered my addiction to crossword puzzles. Daily I take time I don't have to do the one in the *New York Times* and the one in the Syracuse paper as well. Then I make sure I watch *Jeopardy*. I know what these little obsessions are all about. I want the virus not to affect my brain; so these ways are the ones I use to prove to myself that I am still intact.

Yesterday I talked with Mom, Katy, Ellen and Mary Rose. Ellen told me she and Tom have a ticket for me to come to Kansas City to see their new house which sounds great to me—another bargaining time! M.R. has moved to the Provincial House and likes it. Katy's baby is almost due (She thinks it is a girl.), and she likes the sweater I sent. Mother is busy with camp, is planning to fly out to see Ellen's new house and is getting ready to go to Katy's when the baby comes. She is quite worried that Eddie's reserve unit will be activated to go to the Persian Gulf if this conflict continues. More than ever I get the feeling that if people's lives would just settle down a bit, I might be able to tell them about me. Then I know that the reluctance is only an excuse for not wanting to tell them. I could live a long time, and they would worry and be sad for a long time. I guess they have a right to worry about me, and I'm depriving them of that right, but for now, I'd rather get happy letters and phone calls.

I think I *am* doing fairly well. The moments of the day when I think about infection are not representative of my whole life which continues to be good and graced.

September 7, 1990

It's a soft, rainy Friday. We had a fun Labor Day weekend camping on a beautiful lake Barb had recommended. We took the canoe all over the lake and learned how to cooperate with one another in still another way as we navigated the boat. Such amazing quiet! The few small-engine fishing crafts were several miles away; so we heard only the loons.

I felt balanced there. For unsurprising reasons, I was struck by the woods' floor. Huge trees, that must have been hundreds of years older than I could ever be, lay dead, covered with moss and fungi—just giving themselves over. And the decay seemed both gentle and vital.

I think I have said before, perhaps in other words, that I am no fighter, but I love my life, and sometimes the desire to be healthy again hits so hard that it feels as if I have been punched in the stomach by someone three times my size. To think of this disease and me as wagers of a battle leaves me feeling angry, confused and impotent. I suppose it's OK to think of a virus as your enemy, but this thought is rather pointless. Then I can hate myself for getting the virus, for being gay, for hurting my family, for dying early. I can resent the part of the gay population whose sexual behavior was profligate enough to bring the virus within reaching distance of me. I can blame, or even worse, hate the vast majority of individuals in our country for implicitly or explicitly allowing persons like me to die of neglect. But what is the sense of setting up a battleground? I know that love and hope are stronger than all of this hate.

I don't know how to write exactly what I mean. I take my medicine, sleep well and eat regularly because my life is a gift, and I do well to celebrate and honor it. A battle is about survival, not celebration. I don't want to call it *battling* a disease, but I will do everything I can to stay well as my way of honoring the gift of life. Tomorrow, next month, next year might be a matter of life or death, but today is good.

September 20, 1990

It was one year ago today that we found out about Gary's test results. I turned 33 yesterday, and Kate had a little boy (a *big*, little boy) on my birthday. She has always had a way of making my birthday special, but a new life on my birthday is a gift which clearly speaks for itself.

My excitement was a bit dulled by my being sick. After two months, the pain in my leg got to the point where it was impossible to stand up. On Sunday, I was running a fever of 102 degrees and had to take the next three days off from work. By Thursday, I felt somewhat normal again. I was scared about breathing problems, but I had none. (Hell, I'm scared about everything!)

Anyway, my fifth nephew, Maxim, shares my birthday and renews my hope. Thanks, Kate; it was a good birthday, after all.

October 9, 1990

A lot has happened. After all that leg pain near my birthday, I went to the doctor in Syracuse to learn that I had a blood clot in the thigh of my right leg and had to go into the hospital immediately. I spent the whole week in the hospital receiving heparin. Mary Rose had another finger amputated at the same time, and Katy had just had the baby. Mom was rocketing between Binghamton and Ithaca; so I decided one more time against telling anyone. The doctor seems convinced that the blood clot was not related to my HIV status. I'm a bit more inclined to believe him now that I'm out of the hospital.

The trip to North Carolina was a major restorative. I have no words for how sweet it was to see Mike, Maggie, Pat, Jim, Jan and the rest. Pat's baby is beautiful, and he is named for me. I cried when I found that out. At the moment, I feel like a new person with a renewed desire to live well. Dear God, thank you for my friends.

October 12, 1990

I feel good again and am very happy (though quietly so) about that. I get a bit disturbed when I allow myself to start wondering how long I'll feel good. Mostly, however, I'm just grateful for the feeling now, and it's not too hard to let the scarier thoughts pass through.

My GI tract is still in an uproar, but I think that is from the Coumadin I am taking for the blood clot. I have figured out that I do better when I take the medicine twice a day around meal-times than I do when I take both pills at once.

The leaves are past peak, and already it looks wintry outside. I love this time of year. The season makes me grateful for the simple things like a warm place to be, a light against the dark. I bought caramels the other night; so I could dip apples in them. I just want to be home for a while now.

October 13, 1990

It has been a truly awesome autumn, and all day I have been struck by the beauty of everything around me. It's hard to be satisfied with this day only. I find myself asking for more. When I was walking to the car to go to lunch, I heard a clear voice, *my* voice, saying, "OK, OK, I'll go, but I love the life I've been given."

Yesterday the *New York Times* reported the death of Leonard Bernstein. A major part of the obituary was the listing of all he had accomplished in the musical world. On another day, I think I would have been wondering what they will be listing as achievements in my obituary, but that didn't happen today. Quite wonderfully, to the contrary. I am proud of how I have tried to use and appreciate and be grateful for my moments. Growing up I remember hearing that one can easily lose what one doesn't appreciate. If my life on earth is to be taken (and it looks that way right now), it won't be for my lack of appreciation. I hope that in asking for more, I'm making my reason clear: that I'm amazed by what I have already received—the way some persons treat asking for seconds as a compliment to the helping that they have already had. There is no question that I have had a lovely helping that is more than enough. There is also no question that I'd like more. My compliments to the Chef!

October 18, 1990

The local boys' group home burned down last night. The woman who ran the home and three young kids were killed in the fire. The tragedy is very sobering to the staff at the clinic, most of whom have been here longer than I and who have had a fair amount of dealing with both the woman and the kids.

The fire has had the same jarring effect on me that the fire on my street had last winter. Both accidents remind me that most of what goes on isn't about me. On a day-to-day basis, I get wrapped up in confusing, even separating, *my* world and *my* life with life itself. It is something as obvious as the sky, but which, like the sky, I overlook most of the time. I imagine that it is right and human and good that, once in a while these days, I'm able to take something besides myself personally without needing to be the star of the show. Sometimes I think the most wondrous thing about the Creator is that God is able to take all lives, all joys, all sorrows personally—shared and felt but not co-opted. There is just no question—God is on the side of life.

People Magazine is featuring the young woman in Florida who contracted AIDS from her dentist. This issue will sell out because she has the disease through no fault of her own. As I continue to read these days, it seems as if the million or so HIV-infected persons in the U.S. and the ten million in the world have become rather ho-hum because we are, after all, predictable in all respects, including how we got infected, not to mention that the bulk of infected persons (gays, drug users, Africans) aren't exactly high on anyone's list of favorite demographic groups; so we will follow this woman's life and feel compassion because she deserves it (and God knows, she **does.**), and I guess because there is not enough compassion to go around for all of us. I'm no different, of course. I read the papers, watch TV and am bombarded with pictures and numbers that should move me and horrify me; often I just shake my head and say, "Gee, that's awful, isn't it?" Forget fifteen minutes of gore. I think it would be nice if we all got fifteen minutes of compassion to give to someone we think does not deserve it.

October 22, 1990

Sometimes it seems as though my health status is defined more by my problems than by my bloodwork. Getting ready for bed last night, I thought, "I can't be that sick; my problems are too normal—the car, the house, getting ready for Christmas." But out there on the edge of my life, an edge to which I move closer each day, is this slightly more *unusual* part of my life. I can't call it *abnormal* because my situation is one I now share with ten million persons in the world. When will I no longer be able to work? To pay my bills? When will I no longer care? What's going to happen to Gary and me as a couple?

Today is a first—I'm actually finding myself being guided by *Dear Abby!* The reader's response to a man who was HIV+ and wondering whether or not he should tell his family was, to use Abby's words, "overwhelming in favor of his telling them." Now I can at least entertain the idea which was impossible to do not too long ago. Maybe I could tell one or two members of my family, and they could help me decide how and when to tell Mom, or maybe I could tell Mom, and she could help me tell the others. I know it's not fair *not* telling them; they have helped me love who I am. Somewhere along the line, I think they placed some seeds of worth and love in me. To this day, I treasure their love, and yet, I would like to save them the pain. I'm not that powerful, and I know that. I need help with this decision. A little guidance, please. I'm listening.

October 30, 1991

Barb, Gary and I went to see *Long Time Companion* last night. The movie was good—wonderfully funny in parts, although a bit short on character development. Bruce Davison was a real character though, for some reason, they had him die offstage and then cut straight to his memorial service. We were all quiet after the movie.

Last Thursday we went to hear a speaker from Columbia's School of Public Health talk about the AIDS crisis. The speaker was terribly effective, I thought, at making clear to the students that they are *not* free of danger, and that the scope of the disease is now big enough that everyone is affected, if not personally, then economically and socially.

In between those AIDS-fest days, I had a good weekend. Gary's birthday is November 10, and I've decided to get tickets to *Phantom of the Opera* in Toronto. He will love that.

Friday I have an appointment with the doctor in Syracuse. I feel good but have started to dread those visits since they seem always to have nasty consequences.

November 19, 1990

The doctor's visit at the beginning of the month was a pleasant surprise. I had thought I was getting another blood clot in the same leg—no pain but swelling; he said it was nothing, and my Protime was good—no T-4 count this visit, and I am glad of that.

We went to see *Phantom* and had a fun time. The show was more clever than it was great but well worth the trip.

I went to Mass on Sunday and, besides the Liturgy itself, which was lovely and peacegiving, I was moved to tears by all the little kids and all the old people and felt as if some of my sense of order had been restored. I am unsure that there really is such an order; in fact, I'm very aware that I choose to believe in it against my better judgment, but in that choice and with that belief, I have been a happier man. I think the reason for the tears is that I have been getting too wrapped up in my own life, and it was so good to feel a part of something larger. I felt as if I were standing before God with my story, along with the stories of everyone else. And it's a *good* story, far better that it would have been had I written it alone. Far from feeling separate, I feel very connected.

November 29, 1990

I have decided to contact the alternative healing therapist whom Barb had recommended a while back, to start to take vitamins with my other medicines and to be more faithful to the meditation healing tapes each day. It's time for me to take a more active role regarding this infection. I don't know how much any of the activities actually do to help stop the disease's progression, but they do help to make me feel more like a participant and less like a person tied to the tracks listening to the train come. And sometimes it seems possible that I just might last this thing out long enough until someone comes along and invents something that will make a difference.

In today's *Times*, the front page describes the discovery of precisely where on the T-4 cell the virus attacks, a significant enough finding in the sense that it apparently offers some clues to finding drugs that might compete more successfully for the same binding site. On a more practical note, the *New England Journal of Medicine* reported that, on the whole, steroids are useful in treating PCP, even with the accompanying immune-system suppression.

There is an odd sort of helplessness that comes with doing nothing; so I've decided to do what I can. In the long run, my attempts might help nothing, but in the short run, they bolster my attitude and my spirits.

December 3, 1990

The snow has begun. Our first big storm was predicted for this afternoon, and it started two hours ago. Already we have a good ground covering, and it helps to get me into the Christmas spirit. This weekend, I made tremendous advances on my heretofore ignored Christmas list. We went shopping in Lake Placid and then bought our Christmas tree on the way home. Tonight we're going to put up the tree and wrap presents. The snow is spurring us on. Gary loves it even more than I do; the southern boy never takes it for granted.

God, I don't want to be sick. My feelings are so strong from the excitement of the first snow, getting ready for Christmas and the contrast between how I felt in September and how I feel now. It's not so much that I'm afraid of the disease these days as that I just want not to give up anything. On days like these, it seems as if we have chased time back into its cage, and the moments we have are rich indeed. I'm greedy for this life of mine, less because it's the only one I have than because it is the only one I can imagine wanting. One of the readings at Mass Sunday was the parable of the master who goes traveling and gives the injunction to the servants to be ready lest he return at anytime. If he does return, I hope he finds me enjoying the estate because I like it here! I need a bit more trust that whatever is coming my way, I can accept. I'm on a new adventure now (and I like adventures), but I need courage to experience the life that accompanies suffering and dying.

December 14, 1990

Some good developments have occurred. I went to see the alternative healer and liked her very much. She explained the theoretical and philosophical basis of polarity therapy which has to do with getting my energy centers in balance with one another and with the universe. She is going to call one of her teachers who lives in San Francisco and has worked on full-blown AIDS cases to see what specific balancing act is indicated in my case. In addition, she is pursuing a diet designed to boost my immune system. Maybe I can live as long as Linus Pauling, though I think I want not to live *that* long.

The massage that followed my visit with the alternative healer wasn't deep muscle kneading and pounding but far more relaxing, both in process and in the results. I don't know what to make of all this, but I'll be back next week.

The biggest news is that Eddie's reserve unit has been called up to go to Saudi Arabia; he was given only two days notice and will be on his way tomorrow. He'll be employed resettling refugees in the event of a war. The fact that they can do this to a 40-year-old man and my brother is appalling to me and suggests this situation is far worse than they're telling us. At this point, I think Bush's support is falling. I wonder if anyone will support a war over oil involving American men and women or because a tyrant has annexed Kuwait. I think that neither reason is good enough anymore; so maybe the war won't happen.

In any event, I find myself determined once more not to be sick yet. There are too many other things going on. Mother was especially upset about Eddie's being called up and was crying on the phone when she called me.

December 20, 1990

Five days until Christmas! Preparations are virtually finished. This year, I'm going to Utica until Christmas Eve and then returning here for Christmas Day. Gary has to work, and I want to be with him for the rest of the day.

Eddie has gone to Saudi Arabia. His unit left Fort Bragg for Dover, Delaware and flew from there. We have no idea how long he will be gone, but I hope not for long. War is hard for any human being and especially so for someone like my brother who stops a car to move a stranded turtle or to pick up a frightened cat. I wish him home and pray him safety. And I think hard about our country whose immune system broke down long before mine did.

I'm antsy today. I would like to be going on a long trip. The feeling is very much like a desire to leave something behind more than a desire to get somewhere. I used to love driving long distances alone, most often at night. It was wonderful to imagine that it was possible that I might wind up in some unexpected and delightful place by daybreak. I wanted to go to some places just because I like their names, like Biloxi, Mississippi. Sometimes, I feel as if I'm biding my time, as if I'm rooted. I've traveled my own Blue Highways and think I've had enough sense to try to see things as I've passed. Still, today I envision Gary and my packing the truck for a very long trip, plotting our course as we go and returning when it is safe again, maybe never.

December 26, 1990

Christmas 1990 has come and gone. It was better than good; it was great. I left here on Friday for Utica and sort of had Christmas in shifts with Mom, M.R., Kate, Charlie, Rosemary and the kids. There were presents and love galore. As usual, Mom had the house looking and smelling like a Christmas dreamland.

I met for the first time my newest nephew, Max, who shares my birthday. He is a wonderfully happy, laid-back, little baby who just smiles at everyone. Emma Rose is delightful—very smart, I think—and she sat with me in Gram's rocker while I read her stories. I went to the mall with Ed's boys, and we had a great time. M.R. loved her sweater—it was a major hit! I talked to Ellen, Tom and the kids on Christmas morning. The only damper was Eddie's not being there. I hope he felt our love long distance.

Then I returned here for Christmas with Gary, and it was beautiful. Gary had planned dinner. We had goose, a first for both of us and a last for me. We had tons of snow, delivered with a precipitous drop in temperature from record highs Saturday. We visited Barb and Dick in the evening and went to sleep in peace.

January 22, 1991

I am discouraged and tired. My mind is continually wandering, leading me to believe I need a vacation. This has been the situation since yesterday, I think. We are at war with Iraq, a war declared on Eddie's forty-first birthday, and the news, initially about successful air strikes, is now about the use of ground forces. Eddie remains near the front as far as I know. Mother, Rosemary and everyone, myself included, are afraid for him.

Worse, I seem not to be able to get the thought out of my mind that, as a result of my situation, this war and M.R.'s scleroderma, Mom could have, in the near future, three fewer children than she has now. I was obsessed with this idea and asked Barb to make some inquiries from her friend from Veterans' Affairs as to the circumstances needed under which the Army would release Eddie, i.e. family illness. I want to go to someone and say, "Look, you need to send my brother home because my sister could well die one of these days, and I'm going to die probably before long, and my family doesn't know my condition yet. I can't help the aforementioned circumstances, but my brother can be made safer immediately; so do it." This, however, is not the way they do things, and I know it's not the most honest way for me to do things either.

It's funny—I once worried that Gary would soon be sick, and hoped I could take good care of him. Now I'm the one on AZT, and it looks as if I'm the one who is worse. I don't know how to express this part except to say that I was looking at Gary the other night when he was sleeping and thought how *terrible* love is; I think I really mean how *terror-filled* it is. I am used to talking with persons who are lonely and who feel that everything would be better if they could only find someone to love. I found that someone and have to keep reminding myself that the wonder-filled, happy times will outweigh the terror-filled, scary moments.

February 4, 1991

I got a call from the doctor telling me my T-4 count is now 216; so it's time for new measures. We have begun Bactrim DS, a high-strength antibiotic which I take three times a week; it is much simpler than Pentamidine which requires a compressor. I called to make arrangements to see M.R. to tell her about the situation, but she was in Binghamton with another gangrenous finger. I'm going to tell Katy, I think. Why will I not take the risks to freedom? Am I so afraid of rejection? Whom am I protecting?

Wednesday night, I went to have a visit with Father Ray, a local priest. It was a good thing to have done. He felt it would be helpful if I could do some group work with HIV persons and called me later to tell me about a support group that meets in Watertown.

The odd thing is I feel fine right now, even with that count. I don't know what happens from here or when, and that frightens me. I'm looking for a sense of quiet.

February 28, 1991

I have decided to get more serious about some alternative therapies along with the medicines. They may or may not work, but they are worth a shot. Here's what I'm doing. After consulting with André, the therapist, I'm taking lots of powdered Vitamin C—about thirteen grams a day in orange juice. I'm building up to that level because jumping directly into it has caused diarrhea which I can't afford. The Vitamin C is supposed to help me tolerate the Bactrim better, bomb infection agents before they get into my system and somehow help my immune count. That's a very unscientific explanation. In addition, I'm taking lots of beneficial cultures in yogurt and capsule form to combat side effects of Bactrim; so I can keep taking the antibiotics. I'm continuing to see Andrea to get my forces balanced with one another and with the universe. Who knows if this does anything? Who cares? I've found a good local doctor, so that I don't have to keep going to Syracuse, and I'm continuing the AZT, though I can't claim it has done much for me. Finally, I'm praying for the right amount of fight, acceptance and courage like a person who has none, and I'm hoping to wind up with about as much as I need to get by, which is surely fair enough.

Here is the result to date. I feel good. I get a bit tired sometimes, but nothing I can complain about much. I think something is working because everybody has been sick with colds and flus, including Gary, but not I.

In addition, there is the bigger picture. M.R. has had another finger removed but is doing well. Yesterday Bush declared that our objectives in the Gulf War have been met, and troops will start coming home. Perhaps this doesn't apply to Eddie's immediate return, but maybe it does mean that we don't have to worry so much about his getting killed. In any event, I have decided to hold off telling the family. If what I'm doing is working and continues to work, there is nothing to be gained in telling them except pain and worry. I struggle with this all the time and to what point? If I start to get sick, there will be plenty of time to tell them. This is not a fast disease—to many persons' horror.

I have been trying to increase the percentage of time I'm seeing clients at the clinic in an attempt to join in our general revenue-building theme. This has been tiring but largely a good kind of tired.

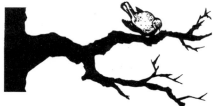

March 4, 1991

A nice weekend! We are watching Barb and Dick's house while they are in Florida, and it has been like taking a vacation. I tried to take Barb's mother to Mass yesterday, but the ice was treacherous, and she decided to stay home. To relieve her anxiety, I took her envelopes to church myself! Father Ray celebrated the Mass, and I spoke with him afterward. A person's kindness means so much; he is a kind, caring man.

I talked with Kate yesterday about planning a surprise fortieth birthday party for M.R. It is tentatively scheduled for two weeks before the scleroderma conference which Mom and M.R. helped to arrange and at which I am the keynote speaker. I volunteered to bake the cake. I have the usual qualms about whether or not I'll be well enough, but that's the story of my life from now on, I guess.

Actually, most of the time now I feel good and calm and happy about my life. It is only when I think ahead and start anticipating the losses that I get off balance. A cover story in *The New York Times* today interviewed five long-time survivors of AIDS; several had their first attacks of KS as far back as 1983 and 1984. I'm not even really symptomatic yet; so I should cut myself a break and think about it less often.

March 18, 1991

What a great weekend we had! On Saturday, I worked on taxes until 5:00 p.m.; then we went to dinner and hit a movie in Potsdam. Thumbs down on *Sleeping With the Enemy.* Gary, who liked the movie (Like most of America, except me, he likes Julia Roberts. *Steel Magnolias, Pretty Woman* and now this, and I'm completely bewildered by her appeal.), even let me have my fun carping about the flick on the way home, and did I ever carp about this one. Boring psycho, boring heroine, boring boy-next-door! A few weeks ago, we drove to Lake Placid to see *Silence of the Lambs,* a movie I thought was truly creepy and effective. Many gay folks, especially those in New York, seem to think it promotes anti-gay sentiments, which appears to me a rather lousy reading of the movie and fallacious in its logic.

Sunday we went to Perth, Ontario, where I found the graves of my great- and great-great grandfathers Noonan. We spoke for a long time to the groundskeeper who regaled us with hilarious Noonan stories. In this village of 9,000, it is still a big name; so the cemetery is filled with my forebears and distant Noonan cousins, persons who live within me and whom I might be more likely to meet sooner than later. Then we hit out for Ottawa and had dinner at the Market before driving home. On both days the weather was about 59 degrees with beautiful, clear, blue skies.

March 25, 1991

I didn't used to understand how persons who knew they were HIV+ could be so surprised and dismayed when they actually developed the disease. Another mystery clarified by experience! I catch myself waiting frequently now for the other shoe to drop, except that it isn't just one other shoe. I think, "OK, what if I get sick soon?" followed by "So then how long will I have?" always measuring and waiting.

Rather against all my better instincts, I have let this infection become the agonizing principle of my life. I watch TV and read the paper looking for news about AIDS. I criticize other news items for disproportionate coverage. (*Disproportionate* is easily defined here; it's what's relevant to *me*!) And I phase in and out of anger and resentment. Some days I feel incredibly put upon to do anything, it seems. Many days I don't feel like going to work, although I'm always better off for having gone. I have this speech coming up for the scleroderma education day and for M.R. and Mom, and I truly dread it, mostly because I'm afraid I'll get sick but also because I'm speaking about how to cope with illness, and I haven't' even told them I'm HIV+. I hate that Mom has to think of two of her children's being sick. Even in all the little things, I find myself making choices as if they really mattered because *I* think they do.

It disturbs me to write all this because I mind that it is harder for me to enjoy life at a time when I should be treasuring the moments most. It's so difficult because, while I don't really feel sick, I'm always exhausted—I think more from projecting future developments than from actual physical activities.

At other times, I think this is all just a sort of letting go which is a normal part of the process. Everything I read admonishes me to fight and never to give up. I certainly don't want to activate my illness or bring on my death; however, it seems that sometimes I care less about things because they really are not so important to me anymore and don't have to be. There is a balancing act going on in my life. I hope I don't drop too many plates.

I want to write, even if the writing might be pure defensiveness (But I think it is not.), that I do a pretty good job most of the time. In fact, most days contain moments of joy that feel infinite. The pain never feels that way. Maybe because I love to travel to new places so much, the idea of resurrection, whatever it is, excites me.

April 4, 1991

Uncle Bunk died during Easter week, and I went to Utica for the wake and funeral. It was much harder than I thought it would be. Mom thought I looked great and happy; she was glad. Part of me was pleased, but the other part wanted to say, "Well, I'm not; I'm dying." I was a pallbearer, probably because Eddie is still in the Persian Gulf, and I felt proud to represent my branch of the family; as the fourth child, I've not done that so much as I would have liked to do it. There was a good feeling of continuity at the wake and funeral—Dad's family, the children, grandchildren and great-grandchildren of Noonie and Dad Noonan. And I like to think of Dad's greeting Uncle Bunk with one of those jokes that only they laughed about, but they laughed for weeks.

Uncle Dick, Aunt Jane, Aunt Tee—they all looked older but good to me. I had to be reintroduced to some cousins I hadn't seen in years and introduced, for the first time, to their children.

There are good things about wakes and funerals; they offer an affirming vantage point. It has something to do with the knowledge that I came from the same roots as these people and will soon be going back. The dead do the living the favor of giving them the chance to get together to pay attention once more to the changing and the changeless. It is strange to watch and think that the next time this crew assembles, the odds are better than fair the gathering will be for me.

A last word on the whole thing—I found myself proud of all these people, proud of all they have given me through the gene line and, to my surprise, proud of what I have done with that.

May 16, 1991

It amazes me how the days pile up. Spring comes hard in the North Country. The weather is warming up, but fitfully, as though winter isn't at all sure it wants to give up control.

In less than three months, I will have been here two years. The time seems much longer. The excitement I remember so clearly was replaced just a couple of months after we had arrived by news of the infection. It's as if I woke up one day and needed to deal with my life from the perspective of one who doesn't have much time left whereas before that day I doubted I was even half way through it.

I finally got a bit of vacation. Gary and I went to Boston and Provincetown, then came back, so that he could cater a sorority party. We then went to Mom's cottage where I finished the dining room table as part of her seventieth birthday gift.

Yesterday I baked the cakes for M.R.'s surprise birthday party this coming weekend. I put them in the freezer and will decorate them when I get to Utica. The cake, along with getting M.R. to Utica, is my part in the surprise gala. After talking with Katy, we came up with the pretext that I would lure M.R. there by inviting her to come and have her picture taken with me and all the nieces and nephews. This arrangement would have the double result of getting M.R. and the kids, who would be all dressed up for the event, out of the house while the others were preparing the party. What I hadn't counted on were all the layers of deception and blundering that had already taken place. John LeCarré couldn't have plotted it in his wildest dreams.

As it turned out, Mary Rose had figured it out. Ellen called to tell her she was coming sometime in May but wouldn't be specific. Then Emma Rose actually told her they were having a surprise party at Grandma's. Even Mom showed Mary Rose a sweet card she had received from Sister Pat on which she had scissored out part of Pat's message. Mom, however, had left in a part that read, "About the party..." When Mary Rose asked Mom, "What party?" Mom said it must have to do with her seventieth, which, of course, M.R. knew hadn't been planned yet because she is planning it! Oh well, I tried, and M.R. still wants to pretend it's a surprise for anyone who still thinks it is. Poor Kate, she was subverted by her daughter, her sister and her mother.

Two weeks from now I have the speech for the scleroderma foundation. The weekend I went to camp, M.R. had two more toes amputated, and her surgeon recommended taking what she has left. I worry sometimes that she and I are in a race to die. However, I worry, not about M.R. and me, but rather about the spectators—Mom, Eddie, Ellen, Kate, everyone.

With all that, I am still very much alive this day. The kids have left school and from my office window, I see nothing but glorious spring. I may decorate M.R.'s cake with edible flowers—the lilacs and apple trees especially are in incredible bloom—or maybe I'll do our five sweetheart roses. This is life at its best, and I am reminded of the old Chinese proverb, *"If I keep a green bough in my heart, the singing bird will come."*

My current bargaining lasts until the beginning of July. God, don't let me get sick before M.R.'s birthday, the scleroderma speech and Mom's birthday. After those events, I'll think of something else.

June 4, 1991

It has been a busy three weeks; I have been gone every weekend. M.R.'s party was a huge success. The cake was a hit; instead of the spring flowers, I decided to go with the different colored roses of our childhood (pink for Katy, coral for Ellen, yellow for Eddie, white for me) with M.R.'s red one on the top since it was her cake and her party! It was a true grown-up party, even with all the kids there—sweet and easy and fun. The four of us did a parody of "Jesus Our Brother" in which each of us sang a verse. Then we gave another performance, called "You'll Be a Sister," based on "You'll Be a Dentist" from *Little Shop of Horrors.*

The difficult part for me was the size of the crowd. I kept being greeted by old friends of Mom and M.R. who told me how good I looked. I felt as if I were betraying my whole family but still felt determined to be problem free. I like to think I'm doing this for them, but I know I'm doing it for myself. It is just easier, I think.

Last weekend, Gary and I decided to go camping and were able to get a spot at Hillside. It worked out especially well because Mom called to say M.R. had to have three more toes amputated Saturday in Binghamton; so we were able to go to see her from the campground, only about forty minutes away.

This was an up-and-down kind of weekend. We had a great time camping, but it was so hard to see M.R. with her poor little foot stitched across the top where her toes used to be. Since she now has no more toes, she jokingly said maybe that would be the end of her problems.

On the way home from the campground, we went to see the

doctor in Syracuse. I had decided that if there were no more clinical decisions to be made based on my T-4 count, I'd rather not know what it was. It turned out that the doctor wasn't going to run the count anyway if I were doing OK on the Bactrim. (I am, thank God.) The next clinical decisions will be made on the basis of toxicity from the drugs or on the development of further symptoms.

This past weekend was the speech to the scleroderma, lupus and arthritis chapters. I kept having this "If they only knew" idea in my head. I mean, many of these persons' illnesses have progressed to the point that you can *see* the disease: the joints in the folks with arthritis, the tightened skin in those with scleroderma, the rashes in the lupus folks. M.R. made it, of course; Eddie had borrowed a wheelchair, and she agreed to be wheeled around. Aunt Ginger made it too, in a wheelchair. I spoke on *Coping, Acceptance and Passion in Illness*, and I know my voice caught a bit in the beginning. I felt a huge sadness for these people's difficulties; they were a kind, even generous, audience. In addition, I felt some compassion that I just know I would not have felt had it not been for the HIV; so maybe a real piece of good in all this is that the virus has expanded my sense of understanding suffering in general, not just my own, and has increased my ability to be compassionate. I even started to smile on Friday night when I was preparing the talk. I was trying to think of an opening and thought about ripping off Father Damien's line, *"We* lepers..."

June 6, 1991

This entry is a continuation of the previous one. The talk went well. It is amazing how scared I was. I mean, two and a half weeks of preparing it, and the night before, I was a real mess. It wasn't only the talk and the fact that M.R. and Mom had asked me to give it. It was being there in Utica in a comparatively high-profile way. The pride they felt in me this weekend only accentuates for me the embarrassment they might feel later on. I know

I'm underestimating them and must feel some embarrassment myself, but it isn't going to be easy. This is a small town where I dated many of the girls and was friends with many of the guys. They know me in a different way, almost as a different person. Then I start to gnaw at myself. Just whom am I protecting by my secrecy? Myself, I know. It's only some faces that trigger such fear and anger in me. (I wish George Bush and Cardinal O'Connor would exhibit some small sense of compassion. Have they lost the message of the Gospel?) Then I have to remind myself that I have met many persons, politicians and Church people included, who personify the compassion of Christ, and that I have seen goodness and kindness more than the opposite during my lifetime. I have had questions over the years about what we have done to *religion*, but my *faith* is deeply my own. And I know I worship a God of mercy and forgiveness, a Jesus of care and concern and a Spirit of truth and integrity.

I am shortsighted and have to keep reminding myself of that. One of the worst things about this infection is that it seduces me to think, and, at times, to judge whether others are good or bad based on my own self-interest, i.e. whether or not they care about and are fighting to save my life. This is a sure route to jadedness and cynicism. Worse, I forget a basic rule of my own. I need to practice trust and good will because the practice is healthful for *me,* and not because it is always fulfilling. Such a practice enhances my own humanity and my faith in the humanity of others.

Time's cover story this week was on the existence of evil. The essay on the inside wasn't so provocative as the all-black cover of the issue was. I'm unsure of the reason I think so. Maybe the reason is that I have asked all the same questions as the article asks. (And, of course, the essay was long on questions and short on answers. How could it be otherwise?) My reaction to the cover was much more visceral. It is a blackness I have *felt.* And I think the reaction is not from the AIDS virus itself, which strikes me as a sort of blunderer, a stupid little organism that doesn't have the sense even to leave its host living. No, the evil, the blackness, is that temptation to think the worst of myself and others simply because *my* life is threatened. Scripture says the only sin is despair. Doesn't it? I agree.

I do have faith in people's goodness, but even more so in the rhythm of life and in God's giving me a place in the circle of love. Sometimes I think of the opening scenes of *Blue Velvet*, when the man has a heart attack as he is watering his lovely lawn in front of his pretty house. The camera goes beneath the lawn, beneath the dead man's feet and the hose still spraying to a close-up shot on the nasty bugs and insects and larvae, just out of sight but always nearby.

It's a neat opening for that wonderfully bizarre movie, but it ignores the beauty of the rhythm of life, of beginnings and endings, gains and losses, joys and sorrows, myself and others. Today I can think that if I don't get all I want, I am happy and excited to have gotten this much.

June 13, 1991

A beautiful afternoon! We are way ahead in terms of nice weather this year—feels as if we have jumped directly from winter into summer. I'm having trouble with the glands in my neck, though. They're not swollen, but they ache a lot, and last week I had some chest congestion. It's strange; I get so focused on the development of symptoms that I forget it *is* possible just to get a cold, the kind that can happen to anyone. I keep centering in on the awful stuff that doesn't happen to healthy individuals, like PCP, KS and toxoplasmosis.

On the whole, I'm still doing well physically. How I'm doing emotionally is often another story. Some of the upheaval comes from the fact that we have decided to renew the lease for another year. It's OK when I remember this home will probably be the only one we'll ever have, but sometimes I get struck by how much I wanted to buy a beautiful, old house to fix up exactly the way we wanted it. My boss recently bought such a house and invited me over last weekend. I was surprised at how jealous I felt. I keep trying to tell myself that we have a beautiful home even if we don't have the deed to it.

The news today mentions a vaccine that has been helpful to HIV+ persons in bolstering their immune systems. The news is very exciting, but it is also a very small, uncontrolled study of limited length. Last night, CNN had a small segment in which they quoted someone's saying that it looked as if, in some individuals, the virus caused fairly debilitating arthritis but in those same persons, full-blown AIDS appeared a less-threatening development. It was strange because Gary looked at me and said rather hopefully, "Didn't you say some of your joints were aching?"

July 8, 1991

Mom's seventieth birthday! Good news and bad news! I read in today's *Times* that many health professionals are suggesting a redefinition of the disease to include anyone with a T-4 count below 200. This change is designed largely to include women, especially those whose AIDS symptoms often do not include KS but do include many other chronic infections. (As the poster says, "Women don't get sick from AIDS; they just die from it.") By this definition, I definitely have the disease. In the good news department, the same article quotes one doctor as saying she has individuals still working full time with T-4 counts of 4, and in the *Voice* this weekend, I read that people typically don't die if their T counts are greater than 50. I try not to pay too much attention to my blood counts because so far, they have had little relevance to the life I am living; besides they scare me.

On the human level, I am doing better than OK. I started working out again and find, rather to my surprise, that I can do it. Maybe I was expecting to crumple up if I lifted weights. It didn't happen.

Over the weekend, Gary and I talked about where we are with the virus and with each other; it's the first good talk we have had in a while, ever since the one in which he asked me if I thought we would still be together if we weren't both HIV+, and we ended up getting angry at each other. The talk allowed us the time really to be together again. I never would have believed that the infection would take such an emotional toll on us, but clearly it has done that.

Mom's birthday is today, and we are celebrating this weekend with a family reunion. M.R. just got out of the hospital from an infection on the spot where the doctors removed her toes last month, and she is better. So, here come the familiar pressures again. I hold off from telling the family, hoping that, if I wait long enough, there will be a new treatment I can tell them about at the same time I tell them I have AIDS. Sometimes I even resent their frequent calls because it draws me closer to them and thus increases the pain they will feel. This is such an ongoing nightmare. Sometimes I get sick of trying to be grateful that I'm at work, not in bed, that I weigh 185, not 85, that I don't have any sores or pneumonia. I'm not really ready to die, but I'm doing it anyway. I'm hoping that, after so many little deaths every day, I will know how to die when the big time comes.

The other night I prayed just to be able to see things differently for a while. My prayer is not just about AIDS, though I'm sure that's the wellspring. The difficulty is that I am now sensitized to suffering, and I see it everywhere: at work, at the grocery store, on TV, on the radio, on the street, everywhere. A few weeks ago, I was listening to Garrison Keillor's radio show, and he brought out Irving Berlin's old clutch-pedal piano. He invited the audience to sing along with "God Bless America," and I just stopped and sang along in the kitchen. I started crying because, for all the time I have loved that song, I've never heard it as a petition before, which it *clearly* is. And it's *clearly* needed.

I want to tell some one in the family now. But whom? Many times I think Mother is the best person. For all the protective impulses we have toward her as our mother, I know she is stronger in her faith and in her love than any of us is. Eddie can't know before Mom because he lives too close to her; M.R. understands me, but she is sick right now; Ellen would have a terrible time being so far away in Kansas City. Katy is my best friend, but she takes things so hard. This is ridiculous. There is no way to pick the right person to whom to hand a dose of severe pain.

August 3, 1991

It has been a long time since I have written. Consistent with the trend of the summer until now, we have been away two weekends between this entry and the last one. Gary and I went camping both weekends and had a wonderful time. We went back to the same lake we had visited last Labor Day. I remembered how much my leg pained then and was grateful not to have that pain this year. I remembered, too, the peace that those huge, rotting trees gave me; it is one spot where the idea of death and life's being part of the same big process doesn't seem like a cliché.

There is no major health news right now. July has gone by, and I didn't get sick. Gary is having a hard time building up the catering business. If I get too sick to work, I don't know what will happen to us financially, but others are managing. I treasure this time of the evening. Gary has gone to bed; I look around the apartment before I go to sleep and, in the shadows and quiet, it looks handsome and peaceful. I won't be buying a home now, but this is home, and I love it. It's so hard to keep a loose grip on things and persons I love so much.

August 29, 1991

Summer is winding down. The college kids are back in town ready to start classes. I feel good, and I sit here amazed at how this infection has gone. In my head, I catch myself thinking that I know how everything is going to go, i.e. I'm going to get sick first; I'm going to stop work first; I'm going to die first. There is, of course, reason to think these things, but in fact, the virus has hit us unpredictably before. Originally, I was sure I would be taking care of Gary. Who knows? That could still happen.

I'm a little scared, but mostly I get tired and worried just thinking about the effect my being ill will have on others. I think about distributing my caseload of work to an already overworked staff; I think about Gary. Will he be able to stay with me if he wants to do that? Will he be able to leave if I die? And of course, my family! I went to camp again this past weekend and saw Mom, M.R., Katy, Charlie and the kids. It was especially nice because Gary wasn't working and came too, and he really enjoyed everyone. I have always been proud of my family and have always wanted my friends to meet each of them. I'm glad Gary is getting to know them better and is comfortable with them.

Mary Rose gave Mother the testimonial birthday book in which we all (kids and grandkids) had written to her what she has meant in our lives. I was amazed to read the passages and think about the family from which I have come. I have always known this, of course, but have never seen a concentrated effort like that of the book. Each person's tribute to Mom was beautifully written—really awesome, not fuzzy like a Hallmark card but so full of sharp, deep, sincere feeling that I cried my eyes out as I was reading the book. The other overwhelming feelings I had were humility and pride to be part of this group of individuals—not that I feel undeserving, just quieted by the idea of how much I share with these people I love so dearly and with whom I am so impressed over and over again.

I want not to intrude on all of this with my news, and somehow I know my family will continue loving me. Sometimes, I'm sure the withholding comes from a real desire to spare them pain.

At other times, the withholding feels childish and selfish arising from my own desire not to share imperfections. I am an important part of this family, and they love me; so there will be pain.

I use the excuse that I will tell them as soon as everything calms down. In a family of our size, do things ever calm down? No, really, to my way of thinking it has been an unusually busy two years. I asked Kate over the weekend whether or not she shares that impression, citing M.R.'s renewed bouts with scleroderma, Eddie's going to the Persian Gulf War, Ellen's moving to Kansas City and her own troublesome pregnancies. She said, "No"; she thinks it is simply people's lives unfolding, following their paths. I'm sure she is right, and this is only my own needed perspective. The trouble is my perspective is the only one I have, but I will wait and pay attention. I still believe that, as the gypsy lady says, all will become clear.

I continue to read and think about Gethsemane as I pray. It is to the point that, as often as I am helped by it, an equal number of times, I feel petulant or foolish, like a child who hopes the chances of getting what he wants increase with the frequency of the request. I guess the difference is that I haven't definitely been told "No" even once; so I keep asking, trying really hard to find the "Thy will be done" part, knowing all along that faith, hope and love are helping me as much as, maybe more than AZT and Bactrim.

Sometimes the whole thing is like taking a very, very long trip. By bus.

September 10, 1991

Today I arrived at work, closed my door and just started to cry. It's Tuesday. Gary left on Saturday for North Carolina to be with his father, whose emphysema has caused him to deteriorate. As I watched him leave for an undetermined amount of time, I felt so alone. Worse, he called last night and is himself overwhelmed at what is happening. His father is much worse than Gary had expected. Gary called an old friend whom he hadn't seen in years only to find out that the friend has AIDS (has known he was HIV+ since 1986), has lost 50 pounds and was in bed with "something he must have picked up." Gary went to visit him and was quite upset. His friend has some KS lesions and is having trouble tolerating any of the antibiotics. He is at home, and his family says he has cancer. Previously he had lived in Washington where, he told Gary, all of his friends are HIV+, sick or dead.

Gary was blown apart and, I think, was looking to me for support. I don't know what kind of job I did. I feel as though I have been kicked in the stomach and feel foolish even saying that. I know that individuals have been watching their friends and loved ones die of AIDS for well over ten years now, and I have known only a few and these few not well. I feel sick at heart for all of them and for Gary and me. Also, I feel very stupid and slow to catch on. Again, it is as though I'm signing up for a club I thought I had already joined. And I don't know how others can witness this senselessness all the time. I guess suffering really does bring us all together because it cuts through the superficial so fast. It is so hard to try to say *yes* to life and death at the same time. Today I'm praying to the *Why-have-you-forsaken-me-Jesus*, hoping he is really out there somewhere for me.

September 19, 1991

Today is my thirty-fourth birthday. Also, the day after to-morrow will mark two years since we found out about the infection. I am tempted to look back through these pages but know I will be embarrassed by some of the things I have written; so I'm passing. Instead, I feel like just summarizing for myself where I am, and what I think I've learned in the past few years.

I have been on AZT for fourteen months, on Bactrim for ten

months; I've been doing Vitamin C and polarity for almost a year. I think these things, each of them so grim to me when I started because they reminded me of how real this disease is, have become as much a part of my day as brushing my teeth. I have improved my eating habits and have become very careful about food preparation. (I haven't had eggs sunnyside-up since I read of HIV infection's increasing the chance of salmonella poisoning.)

I am still at work of which I am quite proud. It seems, if I understand the rules correctly, that I might be able to get disability based on my T-4 count; in fact, if one uses only the count, I probably have had AIDS since last January. However, there is no percentage in it for me not to work and to dwell on having full-blown AIDS. I have learned (and fairly well) how to forget those down numbers and focus more on the fact that I can go about my day-to-day life as well as anyone else. I have established a relationship with Gary that has become fuller and mellower and, to my relief, seems remarkably free of fear (not completely but remarkably). We are together because of love, and we are faithful. I have not told my family yet, a decision with which I am not thoroughly comfortable, but a least right now it is a clear choice, and I know the reason for which I am making it.

I have learned to live with periodic fear, the depth of which had not been part of my previous experience. I have nightmares sometimes about being chased by a small, black thing I can't see. (I wish the dreams of my clients were as easy to figure out.) I have worked with Gary to make our apartment into a home we love. I gave a keynote address to M.R.'s scleroderma group and sang at her birthday celebration. I contributed a piece to Mom's seventieth birthday book and have seen a nephew born one year ago today on my very own birthday. I've worried about money and spent it anyway. Awake and asleep, I have dreamed of lovely things.

In short, I am still here, still alive, and I realize that I love myself and my life. I am stronger and more tender than I ever knew I could be, and I'm grateful to have discovered that. I don't have to be the saddest case in the world to be sad, and I don't have to have a perfect life to be happy—and I sure have had both in full measure these past couple of years. I believe in God, am touched by Christ's humanity, inspired by his divinity and awestruck by his mercy and compassion. I have tried to make something beautiful of my life because it is the only fair way of expressing the gratitude I feel for it.

Still, Gary is gone, and I am lonely. I have settled into a routine and am taking care of myself. I read, play with the cat, make my lunches, meet my clients, take care of the apartment and keep up my friendships.

I received phone calls today from all the family. I think I will celebrate my birthday tonight after all. Thirty-four years are a gift any way you look at it.

September 24, 1991

Gary's father died on Sunday. Gary said it wasn't the awful death the doctor had warned they might have to witness. From what he (the doctor) had said, emphysematics often die in a horrible, literal last gasp, suffocating as they try to take in the air. It wasn't like that for Gary's dad. Gary had taken a break and had gone to town for a few hours, leaving his father with his sister and brother. They were sitting by the pool, and his dad just stopped breathing. Gary was sad but OK when he called. I think I won't go to the funeral, although Gary has made it clear that I would be welcome. I haven't met his aunts, uncles and cousins, and explaining who I am to persons I don't know seems a bit difficult at this point. Instead, I think I'll fly down next week and help Gary with the drive home.

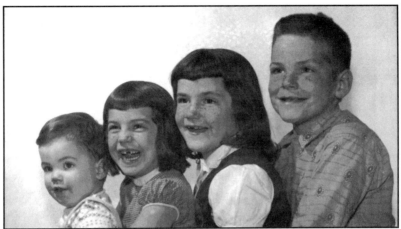

Dick, Ellen, Mary Rose and Eddie—1958

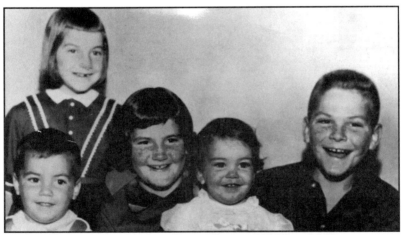

Dick, Ellen (standing), Mary Rose, Katy and Eddie—1960

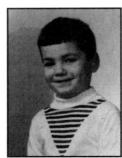

Kindergarten—1962

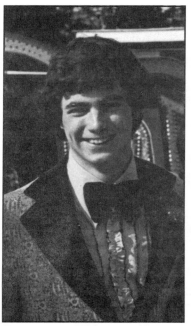

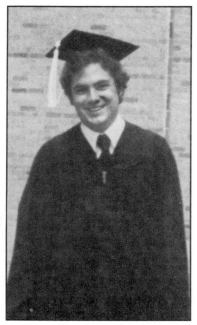

Best man in Eddie's wedding
1975

At Notre Dame graduation
1979

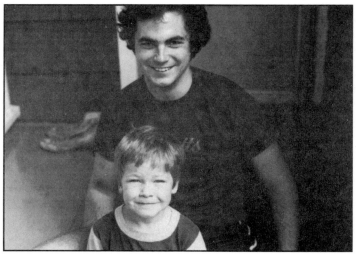

With nephew, Edward—1978

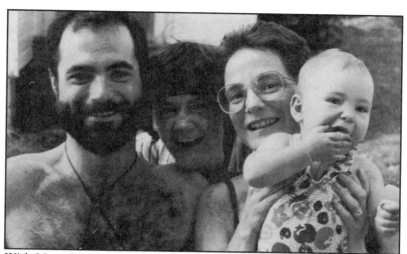

With Mary Rose, Katy, and niece, Emma Rose—1988

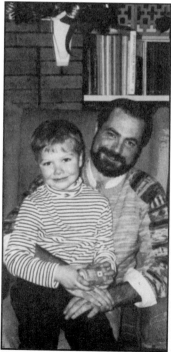

With nephew, Brian—1989

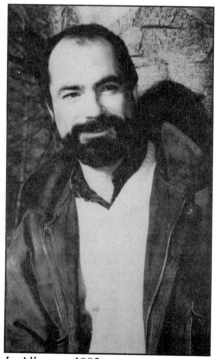

In Albany—1992

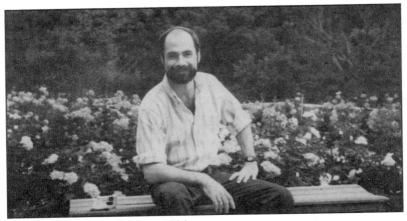

Vacationing in the South—1990

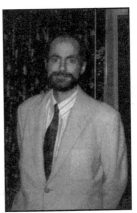

*In NYC to see "Angels in America"
1994—two months before his death*

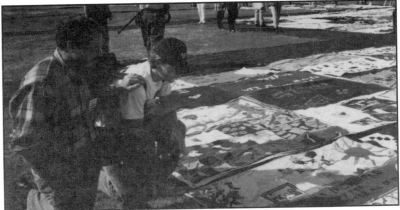

Eddie and Michael at Dick's quilt panel—Washington, DC—1996

October 10, 1991

I didn't fly to North Carolina because Gary is going to stay longer than he had originally planned. He arrived home Saturday, a month to the day he had left. It was strange seeing his face after so long an absence. It was late (about 12:30 a.m.) when he arrived, and after he had taken a shower, we sat and talked a little but really just enjoyed each other. Years ago, I remember going through Cleveland one night on my way back to Notre Dame. A city at night viewed from a train always looked lonesome, or rather, made me feel lonesome. I think the reason is that all I usually saw were the backs of old, brick buildings crowding up to the track and obscuring any view of a skyline. This one night I remember that, right across the parallel rail tracks and through the rain, I could see into the one window that was still lighted at 4:00 a.m. It was several floors up, but because the train was on a bridge, the room was straight across from my line of vision. And this little place looked like someone's home. I could see pictures on the wall over a bed and an old-fashioned, pole lamp. I remember wanting to know who lived there, and why they were up at that hour of the morning. The train was moving slowly, and the window was far enough away that it took a few seconds to pass from my view. I saw no one inside, but I remember wishing happiness to whoever lived in that little room overlooking the train.

That view came back to me as I sat across from Gary in the apartment on Saturday night. In my mind, I saw our house from the outside, one lighted window burning against all the others. If anyone passed by and wondered what was happening beyond that lighted window, it was just two persons' being company to each other in a home they had worked hard to make lovely and warm.

October 15, 1991

Mike came up from North Carolina for the long weekend, and we had a wonderful visit.

My leg started hurting last Wednesday night on the inside of my upper right calf; it hurt only when I got up or sat down. The pain got worse on Thursday but leveled off on Friday which certainly is a comment on the analgesic value of having friends visit. The pain is back now at the inside bend of my knee; so I think it is another blood clot. I was quite discouraged last night because I want not to return to the hospital again for IV Coumadin. I have to figure out what I'm willing to do and then get more willing to do it. And maybe it's not even a blood clot.

October 28, 1991

My leg cleared up before I went to the doctor; so I don't have to feel guilty about not taking a suggested treatment. We turned back the clocks on Saturday night. As I write this entry at 4:30 p.m., the sun is setting over the treetops, and it will be dusk by 5:00 p.m. It has been Indian summer this whole past week, and I hate to see the early darkness come. With the short afternoons and the frost in the air, one can feel winter's coming on strongly. I am excited already about Christmas but not about winter this year.

We had a wonderful weekend with the last of the warm weather. John and Raymond invited us down to the costume party/fund-raiser for the AIDS organization of which they are a part. Gary had called a costume company in Schenectady and reserved the Union/Confederate troop costumes for us, and they were really authentic ones. We had a ball. John and Raymond have a crowd of friends, all of whom were wonderful at making us feel welcome.

We stayed overnight and had Sunday brunch with them and some other friends. Our costumes won the two awards at the party; that was actually quite embarrassing because they were rentals, and many other guests there had put tons of time and work into their own getups. I like these guys a lot and hope we will continue to see them.

November 8, 1991

The first real snow of the season is falling outside my window. In a few months, I may be tired of it, but right now it is new and exciting, and the air smells like Christmas.

I find that I like counting back since the last time I wrote—eleven days. It is as though I have just survived a quintuple somersault on a trapeze. Of course, the truth is that I've simply been living my life. Still, when I watch the snow and realize I still feel good, the feeling *is* thrilling.

I went crazy over the weekend buying wool for sweaters; the ones I made last year were such a big hit. I have started an Icelandic pattern in mohair for M.R. for Christmas, and so I'm covered with fuzz. I bought the same kind of yarn in purple for Kate, and I want to find something pretty for Ellen, too. I hope I can finish them all by Christmas. I'm ripping through M.R.'s quickly, and Kate's looks rather simple; so maybe there is a chance I'll succeed. Also, I bought some off-white and blue yarn from Gary and Brian (from their own sheep), which I think I'll use to make myself a sweater. It's wonderful, warm stuff.

I had a doctor's visit on Friday. No news which, in my case, is definitely good news. He measured my leg to make sure there was no clot and feels that I have had relatively few side effects from the AZT. He could feel my spleen but thinks that's not a problem. I had a flu shot and a pneumonia shot, and that's about it for now.

I talked with M.R. over the weekend. She has new doctors in Albany; so she doesn't have to keep returning to Binghamton. They want to do a kidney biopsy, but M.R. is reluctant. She has had two in the past; one was quite painful, and both showed some kidney involvement from the scleroderma. She isn't convinced

the biopsy is worth it but will decide this week. Again I find myself amazed by the persons in my family. Maybe it is a family just
like everyone else's; no, I have seen enough to know this just
isn't true. Once again, I hope they will all understand my not
telling them about the HIV; I know they love me and am strength-
ened simply by that knowledge. I spoke with M.R. again on Saturday. I understood better, but not in a way I can articulate well
here, the old idea of offering up one's pain to enable it to be
redemptive. Maybe it's just the idea of being challenged to find a
value in all human experiences, especially the hard ones. In any
case, I'm not in a lot of pain these days, but I *do* get scared. I'll
try to offer that. Dear M.R., God is showing me to myself through
you right now, and I like what I see. Thank you.

November 22, 1991

Since I last wrote, Magic Johnson announced his infection
and, for about a week, the general population went nuts. On the
whole, though, I think the results were good, and people were
compassionate. Also and predictably, the news media quickly got
wrapped up in how he got the virus, and he was called upon to
assure the public that he was heterosexual. The usual backlash
developed criticizing his promiscuity, although I imagine it would
have been worse had he announced that he was gay. Ironically,
at the same time, Wilt Chamberlain published his autobiogra-
phy claiming that he had had sex with over 2,000 women.

Tony Richardson, who directed *Tom Jones*, died of AIDS
last week. *Beauty and the Beast*, the Disney flick, is coming out
this week to rave reviews; the lyrics are by Howard Ashman, who
died of the disease last spring. All of these supposedly big developments are drowned out by the honking of the geese as they
pass by overhead. I imagine their voices to be a derisive com-
mentary on the nonsense that goes on below—humans struggling to be human.

I still love people as much as I've ever loved them, but I hope I'm expecting a bit less of them. I have been and probably will continue to be angry about the lack of response to this disease but am forced to admit that even I can't scrape up the same compassion as I have for the starving children I see on TV. Being angry separates and tires me. Some say anger will keep me alive longer but, like that new drug for CMV infections of the eye, it's at the cost of a miserably protected existence. No, I have to find a better response for myself. I want not to be sick in spirit too.

It is 4:55 p.m. in late November. As I look outside my window, I can see the last of the winter light draining from the sky. Today I draw my comfort from a rhythm that is better than human, and I pray that visions of all that is good and beautiful in my life will carry me through the fear and the pain.

December 31, 1991

It has been over a month since I've written. There is a bit of news. One of my classmates from Binghamton has applied and been accepted for a job here at the clinic. Initially, I thought my lack of excitement was due to a feeling of competitiveness. Only afterward did I realize that she comes back into my life from the "other side." She knew me pre-gay, and I'm not really interested in updating her. Even worse, I find that I am embarrassed about my HIV status. Not ashamed, not guilty, embarrassed. I think the reason is that, while I don't consider my infection to be the kind of mistake many might think, it *is*, nonetheless, a mistake of lousy judgment. It's natural enough, I think, to be embarrassed by such mistakes and to want to keep them private. Life is usually more forgiving on this respect, though. It makes me uncomfortable that, at some point, my judgment (of which I'm usually quite proud) will be open to question by every one who hears my story. I want to control the speed of information about my life, but I won't be able to do that.

This thinking is more than a little irrational and, like most things I have worried about in life, will not be so painful as I think. For one thing, I never have had any control over what people say or think; for another, time and again, people's goodness and kindness have been made apparent to me, and they will be again, I trust; so I will be OK about this. Eventually.

I spoke with Maggie a couple of weeks ago. She had just discovered that she has inoperable breast cancer and was about to order a wig anticipating total hair loss from the radical chemotherapy she has already begun. Her chances are not good, but they aren't negligible either. She is frightened, and we had a good conversation. I'm so glad she didn't hold back the news on my account. (Maybe I shouldn't hold it back from my family either.) There really is no point in feeling sorry for either one of us—and I told her so laughingly—because we aren't sad cases. And death isn't sad; it's normal and natural. What isn't quite so normal is knowing that you're likely to die much sooner than you had expected, but even that is far from unique. No, Maggie and I aren't sad because we both know something about happiness and gratitude simply for having life itself. We may not know much about death, but we both have learned a lot about life. I'm thinking we can learn about death in the same way—by experiencing it.

I saw a repeat of William F. Buckley's interview with Malcolm Muggeridge the other day. Muggeridge talked a lot about ways of coming to know God, the important dialectical relationships between doubt and faith and the directly proportional relationship between belief and humility; the latter led him to conclude that, if he approaches God following death, it will be "in quite a craven fashion." I found myself nodding and came away thinking, "Maybe I am on an OK track."

Christmas was wonderful. Gary and I celebrated together on Christmas morning and then drove to Utica where we stayed until Friday. Everyone was there—Mom, M.R., Eddie, Rosemary and the boys, Ellen, Tom, Jess and Thomas, Katy, Charlie, Emma Rose and Max. We had our caroling and poetry at the table, as usual, starring Mom and me.

It's New Year's Eve. I resolve to quit smoking, to be faithful to the Vitamin C, to take an aspirin every day, to get moderate exercise, to be less angry with myself and others, to be a better lover of those I love. Bring on the New Year. I'll try to keep my hair combed.

January 6, 1992

Yesterday I invited Jack over to the house. Gary had to cater a party and was gone all day. I was home with nothing pressing to do; so I figured this would be a good time to call him. I felt bad because the doctor had asked me in early December whether or not I would be willing to call Jack. Time got away from me during the holidays. Actually, I think there was a bit of avoidance; he is much sicker than I am.

Jack came over within a half hour of the call and stayed for five hours. I think I like him, and I know I respect him. He has known for a few years that he is positive and lives in a tiny, one-room apartment with no car. He does have family nearby and plans to move in with them in the spring.

Jack has lost 50 pounds this past year; he hasn't had PCP or KS but has had lots of debilitating infections and fevers, especially in the GI tract. He has frequent headaches as well and today is getting back the results of bloodwork which he hopes will identify whatever he has that has kept him down for the past few weeks.

We sat there talking about many things, but he always drifted back to what is happening to him physically, not in an annoying or self-pitying way though. I think we were sort of comparing ourselves with each other. He would ask, "Has that happened to you yet?" and generally speaking, the answer was, "No," i.e., I haven't had thrush; my weight is stable; I don't take Pentamidine because I'm tolerating Bactrim, etc. I even found myself exaggerating a bit in case there should appear too great a distance between us physically, a distance that might upset or distress him at the present time. He is much further along than I am, I think.

February 7, 1992

A full month between entries. January was busy. Aunt Ginger died in her sleep two weeks ago yesterday. I went down to the funeral. She had been sick for a long time, but her death was still a surprise. It was hard to see Mom grieving her sister—Mom is the big sister and, I imagine, feels toward Aunt Ginger and Aunt Ann the way M.R. feels about Katy and me—and I know that is a *very* strong love. Also, I kept thinking of the new sadness Mom will have soon. I love you, dearest Mother.

Mary Rose gave the eulogy, and I did the readings at the funeral Mass. Eddie and Katy were there, but Ellen couldn't get in from Kansas City; I know the distance frightens her at times like these. It was a weekend about connections, and so, in the end, I felt better. As much as I realize that my sickness will cause the people I love great pain, I looked around and realize that I come from "good stock," that my life's struggles and joys are important to these persons, and that they have shown again and again their love for me. They will keep doing that; so I trust we'll make it through. I come from people with faith and passion and strength. I know they will help to let life pass through me, so that I can go on.

February 13, 1992

Tomorrow I fly to Kansas City to see Ellen, Tom and the kids on a frequent flyer Tom gave me. I'm flying out of Montreal, and I'm so excited to be taking a trip I never thought would come.

I talked with M.R. last night. She is at the convent in Binghamton and had part of another finger removed. Although she called it a "small part," I could tell she was in pain. I told her how good I think she has been about the scleroderma over the years. I wanted to say more—that I get great strength from the fact that I don't have to look any farther than to my own big sister for example and inspiration on how to live with hard things. Actually, in other ways, Mother, Eddie, M.R., Ellen and Katy all serve this function for me. We are strong, funny and, I think, graceful people. I didn't say those things to M.R., but I will do that sometime.

March 2, 1992

I had a terrific time in Kansas City with Ellen, Tom and the kids. Their house is what I would call a mini-mansion, and Chère has made it warm and homey. Tom is a natural tour guide, and I think I saw most of the city in a few days. The kids are funny and smart and completely hospitable. The trip couldn't have gone better, and I felt fine.

March started over the weekend. Some strange weather pattern occurred when it was fifteen-twenty degrees below zero during the day and warmed up enough at night to snow. The result is that we have more snow at once right now than we have had all winter. I want spring to hurry up. In fact, I'm praying that God will hurry all the good things along, and I wonder whether or not God is hearing any of my prayers. Then I remind myself that God is right here inside me. I hope he likes it.

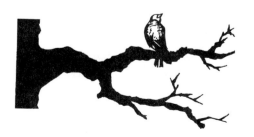

March 23, 1992

Spring officially began over the weekend, but winter's grip on our area continues to be unrelenting. It was eight degrees this morning. I read in the *Times* that this was one of the warmest winters on record, but I can't imagine that this is true locally. In my mind, I am constantly driving to some place warm. Originally, I had planned to drive down to Mississippi in April, but now I don't know. I'm getting concerned about money these days. There are things for which I'd like to save. Some of those things are about living; others are about dying. The lady next door has a small trailer for sale that I think would be great fun for our camping trips. Sometimes I think we might need a better computer, especially if I get sick. I could type papers for students, and Gary could use it to facilitate managing his business. I'd like to buy another car. And I'd like to pay for my funeral.

I find that life requires a regular commitment from me that I don't always feel like making. I have to stop guessing about how much time I have left; it keeps me from finding reasons to do needed things. Balance becomes harder than ever. To save or to spend? To change or to accept? To engage or to withdraw? I try to be quiet and listen. I can do better.

March 31, 1992

Finally, some spring weather! Traces of snow are still on the ground, but the skies are clear, and the temperature is nearing 50 degrees. It is very distracting to be at work when it seems as though life is going on outside my window.

We went to an auction this past weekend, and I picked up a beautiful, walnut Victorian table, a round oak table and a Larkin dresser. They all need a little work. The dresser is painted white, and will need to be stripped. Given the break in the weather, what I want to do is to go home, pull the new pieces outside and begin working on them. Actually, I used a heat gun on the drawers last night to get the paint off—never my first choice but OK if I'm careful. Of course, I hear a little voice in my head saying, "Hurry, hurry," and urging me to get these pieces finished. This is a fairly common feeling these days, but is at least a whole lot better than the voice that says, "Don't bother." I hate that one.

The Academy Awards were last night. Howard Ashman, who died of AIDS a while ago, received the "Best Song" award. How odd it is, I thought. Last year I rooted so heavily for Bruce Davison to win a supporting-actor award for playing an AIDS victim in *Long Time Companion*. This year, I watched as an award was given to a real-life guy already dead from the virus. It gets more real all the time.

No doubt partly as a result of the telecast, I dreamed last night that I was looking in the mirror and, on tilting my head back to shave, saw these incredible, dripping tumors, running from ear to ear. I woke up immediately and had to calm down a bit before I could get back to sleep.

April 3, 1992

I was paying bills last night when Mary Rose called to tell me she is having the rest of her little finger removed today. She is, of course, good about it, but very sad and tired of parts going rotten and needing to be cut out or cut off. We talked about her decision regarding whom to tell and when, something she has to think about every time she has this done, and something in which I am very interested. She has told Mother, Kate and me. She would rather tell Ellen and Eddie after the surgery. Ellen is so far away and would want to be with M.R., and Eddie gets so worried. M.R. figures it's easier for them to hear her voice after it is all over. The trouble is that *all over* for her and *all over* for me mean two different things at the moment.

Kate called afterward, and we spoke for quite a while. She is going to try to get to Binghamton on Sunday depending on how

M.R. feels by then. Her pregnancy is going fine. Emma Rose, who is now five, is very opinionated about the baby's name; she thinks she can't love a baby girl named *Rebecca*. Apparently, *Brendan* is the only satisfactory boy's name. What wonderful kids my brother and sisters have! I'm so eager to see how they turn out, and somehow I will, even though it may be from some unknown and undiscovered place.

We are having Raymond and John up for the weekend, and I'm thrilled. They called earlier in the week and asked to come. Jim is coming up at the end of the month. I'm not going to get out of here for a trip this month, but the company is the next best thing.

I have a wartlike thing on my lip and another coming on my cheek. The doctor says maybe he can burn them off. I feel like a piece of furniture whose finish is wearing off, and I guess it's from the inside out.

Earlier on in this disease, I think I was better at intellectualizing the situation. Now I find myself happier with the simpler things. I'm glad that my eyes work even though they itch. I'm happy that I made it through another week at work even though I'm tired and can't get a grip on the paperwork. And right now, I just want to get those tables refinished and set up.

April 22, 1992

Finally we really have spring. Temperatures are in the 60s and 70s and, although it's rainy, the air feels wonderful.

Last night I dreamed I had a child. He was about one year old and beautiful. I don't know who the mother was, but I was separated from her. In the dream, I had to go to Connecticut to pick up my son from his unnamed mother. What I remember most distinctly was driving with the child, my child, sleeping in the car seat next to me. I would stop at rest stops to take care of him, feed him, change him, the whole bit; I was on my way to

Utica to show him to his grandmother. And I felt so good at the job, as if I really knew what I was doing. When I woke up, I felt as though I *had* had the experience of being a parent, not as though I had had a dream. The experience was so real that if anyone had asked me whether or not I had any children, I could have answered with complete honesty, "I did once," not "I dreamed I did once." I wasn't sorry to see my real life on waking; the dream felt like an addition or maybe a complement to my real life, a bit as though one had taken a vacation from a job he really loved. When he returns, he is glad he went but isn't sorry to return.

I planted roses on the sunny side of the house yesterday. I've finished one of the tables I had bought at the auction, and it looks great in the hall. The other table and the dresser are well on their way.

May 15, 1992

I write at the end of another workweek, staring out the window, waiting to get outside; it is so beautiful.

I'm staying home this weekend after having gone away for the past two weekends. Two weeks ago, Gary and I went to visit Katy and Charlie in Newfield. We had fun. It was the first time I had been to their new house, and it is beautiful—up on a hill, looking across a valley to a beautiful ridge. They are a wonderfully sweet family and very easy to visit. We walked the incredible gorge at the park and hit downtown Ithaca. Katy looks amazingly good considering the baby is due in six weeks. They have a boy's name picked out—*Brendan John* (*John* after me), but are juggling girls' names and seem to think it's a girl. Mary Rose thinks that Kate knows whether it's a girl or a boy.

Last weekend, I went to Utica for Mother's Day. We had fun. M.R. came from Albany, and Mom's two childless children went with her to Mass and then to brunch. I brought my pipe clamps to help Mom work on some good dining room chairs she had bought. I brought back a terrific armchair, a lamp, some towels, a candlestick and a beautiful carving set—all items Mom had picked up for me at various sales. I brought Mom a dozen roses which looked lovely next to the flowers Katy and Ellen had sent and the plant Eddie had brought. Mary Rose is no fool—she brought Mom a bottle of scotch from New Hampshire. You can't drink roses.

I went to the doctor's Friday before I left for Utica. I had complaints this time—the noticeable growths on my face and a rash on my leg. He said the growths really are warts, and acid will burn them off. Initially, we are treating the rash on my leg with a cortisone cream. The rash, located on the back of my left calf, is quite blotchy and very itchy. The doctor's idea is that it could be one of two different types of dermatitis or the remote possibility of a KS lesion. If the initial treatments don't work, he will suggest a puncture biopsy. I think it's not a KS lesion.

A bit more ominous is my bloodwork which shows suppressed everything—red cells, white cells and platelets. Of course, these side effects result from both AZT and Bactrim. The counts are not low enough to discontinue the medications, and the doctor wants neither to add nor to substitute DDI at this point. Also, he took some blood for a T-4 count which I haven't had tested in a long time. While taking it, the doctor told me he has a friend whose T-4 count has been less than 30 for three years and is in better shape that one would guess.

I feel OK except for the rash and occasional fatigue. Now I need a nap at work, and every time I have a free hour, it's a tough choice between a nap and paperwork. Guess what gets chosen? Today, about the only other thing I can say is that I'm living. That's fair enough.

June 10, 1992

It has been a while since I last wrote, and happy things have been happening. We had a visit from Jim over the Memorial Day weekend. We picked him up in Ottawa and took him all around our area, including Lake Placid and Montreal.

Kate hasn't had her baby yet. I talked with Mom this weekend; she said the doctor said the baby is seven and one-half pounds at this point, and he wants it not to get much bigger than eight and one-half pounds for Katy's sake. Thomas invited me to be his confirmation sponsor next year in Kansas City, and I was so touched. He is thinking of taking *John* for his confirmation name. Also, I began immediately to experience the same old worry as always when I commit myself to something in the future. A bit closer on the timetable is Ellen and Tom's visit to camp, which is supposed to happen June 20. I'll go down to see them for certain.

We have put in a whole cutting bed around the roses. Also, we planted dahlias, carnations, snapdragons, coreopsis and lupin. We don't really know what we're doing, but we're doing lots of it. I go out often to weed and water, prune and fertilize. In addition, we have a little patch in back with tomatoes, peppers, broccoli and herbs. I'm more excited about the flowers, but Gary likes the vegetables.

I finally finished my will and my healthcare proxy, speaking of vegetables!

August 24, 1992

Barb told me that a number of people at work are concerned about how I look and hinted strongly to her that they had suspicions about my HIV status. I guess I have been looking thin and drawn. We talked a bit and decided that, while I was in North Carolina visiting Mike, Barb would let my friends at the clinic know. I'm letting Barb tell them because, as with my family, I just can't bring myself to do it. When I called Monday night, Barb had, indeed, hit everyone. It is interesting that, in the case of many of the women, Barb was only confirming a suspicion they had already formed, based on their observation of me. The men, on the contrary, were, according to Barb, entirely without suspicion and rather blown away by the news.

After five days in North Carolina, which were refreshing and restorative and which preserved, perhaps saved, my sanity, I realized I wanted to come back home. When I arrived, there was a lovely plant waiting for me from the folks at work. They were then and continue to be wonderful to me. I, on the other hand, continue to be uncomfortable with people, even those to whom I consider myself close. It's my problem; they have welcomed me back saying little but expressing a very sincere and warm concern that is both heartening and moving to me. I am a lucky man; nearly every one in my situation knows stories of persons who have lost their families, their friends, their jobs, their minds.

One week ago today, I had an appointment with the doctor to go over the results of my bloodwork, and my T-4 count was 50—not good news. He suggested it was time for me to go to the University of Vermont to hook up with an infectious-disease man there and largely to talk about where to go with my medication regimen. Also, he suggested that I call the local person who works as the St. Lawrence County representative to the AIDS Task Force in Syracuse. We then started a regimen of Amoxicillin to treat what was suspected to be a nonhealing staph infection on my left cheek.

That weekend, I went to camp because Katy was there with Elizabeth Kathryn who had been born June 22. I hadn't made definite plans but hoped the opportunity would come to tell Katy. Late Saturday night, Kate and I were sitting and talking; everyone else had gone to bed. Somehow, finally, and I don't remember how, the conversation turned to AIDS, and Kate said, "You're not worried about it?" I paused and thought a long time and then said, "No, I'm actually not too worried about it." She said, "But you have been tested, and you're negative, right?" I: "I didn't say that; I said I wasn't worried." Her eyes seemed to be getting very big, and I had trouble looking at her, sitting there nursing her beautiful new baby. She said, "Don't tell me what I know is true." I couldn't do anything but nod. She came and sat next to me and, except for one brief moment, stayed calm. We talked a few more hours until around 3:00 a.m.. As I left the next morning, I saw her standing with Mom, M.R., Charlie and the kids and trying not to cry as I pulled away.

Dear Kate, you have always been one of the sweetest joys in my life, and I love you so much.

I went to Burlington on August 5. The doctor there suspects that I am now resistant to the AZT and thinks I should add DDI to the mix. He favors the combination of AZT and DDI to DDI alone and prefers DDI to DDC because of his experience that the neuropathy, a major side effect of DDC, occurs more frequently than pancreatitis, the major side effect of DDI. He thinks the sore on my face is not herpetic, but he wrote a script for an antibiotic just in case.

I think I forgot to mention that we bought a van in which to go camping and used it for the first time during the week of August 11. I'm trying to insert something fun here in between descriptions of my medical state. Also, I'm exercising again—lifting weights and trying to pick up the steps of a country-western dance video. I've been careful about my diet, especially about eating three, decent meals; breakfast has always been a challenge for me. My sleep is good, and I'm using relaxation tapes quite frequently. I've gone decaf, too—a major step.

I followed the doctor's recommendation about contacting the representative from the AIDS Task Force. She came over, and we did a needs-assessment type of interview. She was extremely nice, rather young. Her caseload is small, and I am the only one with my own transportation and private insurance. I obtained some information about how to apply for Social Security Disability when the time comes. I have qualified medically for several months, but I intend to keep working as long as I can. The clinic has been wonderful on this score; they have offered to let me be part time if I need to be. It is a kind, thoughtful offer because we are really not set up for that.

I don't know what to make of all this. My bloodwork suggests that the virus is continuing to work its relentless devastation on my system; I have a sore on my face that leaves me very self-conscious, but it is getting better. Many more persons now know, which, while somewhat uncomfortable for me, is, on the whole, a good thing. Katy knows which means more than I can ever say. And I have a lovely, new niece who doesn't know yet how lucky she is to have been born into our family; her uncle knows, though.

It has taken me a few days to update this journal, and I'm not sure of the reasons for which I want to put in all those details-maybe because it's my life, all of it, and I understand that better than I once understood it. Important things should have witnesses, and my life is an important thing; so I write. And I know I am graced because of the ability to express the sentiments of a grateful heart.

September 9, 1992

I am trying to get back into the habit of writing more regularly. We are moving into fall without ever having had a summer this year. But then, I was a bit preoccupied this summer and didn't pay much attention to the weather.

Mike came up from North Carolina this past weekend which included Labor Day. We had a good visit, and he noticed the comfortable routine into which we have slipped. I'm always busy doing small chores and value, more than ever, time alone. This is particularly difficult for Gary who continues to be asymptomatic, but our weekends are always so filled with people. Next month,

Gary, Raymond, John and I are going to D.C. to see the AIDS quilt before it is separated into regional pieces. Julie and I have made a regular thing out of dinner on Wednesday nights. I talk with Mike weekly and with my family as frequently, and I tend to hear from Kate a few times a week. And these are just the regulars.

October 29, 1992

How long I have been meaning to get to this journal! I left the last volume in the van, and I'm not clear about when I last wrote. I think it was in late August or early September.

I have been happy and busy. I'm eating well, sleeping well and have gained the thirteen pounds I had lost during spring and early summer.

On September 19, I turned 35. It has been three years since I learned of the infection and I think four to four and one-half years since I got the infection. My birthday coincided with a camping trip, the last of the season, and the Albany guys brought along a cake. My sweet tooth has not gone into remission. I ate more of the cake than anyone else ate and was a regular pig about being sure I kept getting big, pink frosting roses.

On October 12, I had another follow-up appointment with the doctor here in Potsdam. Apparently, my chemistry values are highly consistent with a diagnosis of a healthy person, but my blood-cell counts continue to fluctuate—mostly abnormal. I don't pay much attention to them as long as I feel good. I just get up every morning, check myself out, declare myself fit enough to have a day and get on with it. I'm anemic and have to be careful; on rare occasions, I feel as if I am going to fall asleep from a sudden exhaustion wherever I am. This propensity is usually controlled by getting a regular eight hours of sleep and a periodic nap. I can't say that I have actually dropped off to sleep, and God knows, some of our meetings provide all the inducement anyone could need; so I guess I'm OK.

We have added Acyclovir for herpes and Bacitracin prophy-lactically for TB to the mix of meds I am already taking—AZT, DDI and Bactrim. I notice that my skin seems to be suffering; it's very dry and itchy but certainly tolerable. I believe most of these prescriptions can cause pleuritis and skin problems over the long haul, but I still feel very lucky that it isn't much worse.

About the only complaint I have comes from the wartlike growths in each corner of my mouth. We continue to address these by weekly freezing with nitrogen, and the treatments have reduced them to a manageable size. Also, I try to keep my mous-tache longer at the corners. It works usually, but the last time I saw Mother, she told me to wipe the corners of my mouth to get the food off. If I can't do any better, I'm considering having rhine-stone studs planted at each corner. In this age of body piercing, I might start a trend that has already moved from ears to noses to navels to everywhere else. On the other hand, rhinestones in the corner of my mouth probably would make that section of my face look like the grill of a '69 T-Bird. I'll stick to the nitrogen.

On Columbus Day weekend Gary and I went to DC with the Albany guys to see the quilt—all fifteen sad and sweet, lovely and loving, and even, I think, holy acres of it. I am wholly inad-equate in trying to describe the weekend and its effect on me. The quilt itself was every bit as awe inspiring as the Washington Monument in whose shadow it was laid out, and certainly more poignant. I like Washington. I'm always thrilled by the memori-als and the monuments. I actually feel a part of something great—just being an American. A bit to my surprise, that feeling was enhanced, not diminished, by the quilt.

There was anger in me, too, sometimes bitter enough to taste, and an enormous sadness, but my overwhelming experience was one of identity and community. There were many families and many children, mothers and fathers, every emotion on display and plainly readable on beautiful faces. The same wonderful variety was present in the panels of the quilt itself. I saw partners straightening out the wrinkles in the panels of their beloved dead, and I heard brave mothers reading from an incredibly long list of victims, often concluding with a sweet remembrance of their own sons and daughters. And I felt as intensely alive as I ever have felt even as I thought of my own death. There was love for myself, gratitude for my own life and for my family—knowing that their love will memorialize me—and a greatly eased fear of my death. Too, there was, a strange sense of belonging with both the living and the dead.

November 19, 1992

I am trying to recommit myself to writing in this journal. Thanksgiving is a week from today, and I have much for which to be grateful. Right now, the plan is to go to Latham and spend the day at the Provincial House with M.R. and Mom.

Kate came to visit this weekend and brought Elizabeth Kathryn who has gone from being an infant to a real little girl with an amazing personality. She is five months old and spent the visit smiling and laughing. Actually, that is mostly the way Katy and I spent the weekend as well. Apart from the hilarity, I gave her copies of my important papers: my will, my healthcare proxy, my list of insurance policies and creditors, and individuals to be notified when I die. Kate asked if I would consider moving to Ithaca at any point. She and Charlie are thinking about moving into town and are looking at a house with an apartment. It is a wonderful offer and a surprisingly comforting one to me. Ithaca is nice; I would be closer to the doctors; best of all, I would be nearer to my incredible sister, my dearest friend.

I'll continue to think about the offer, though for now I'll stay in Potsdam and live the life of a true son of the North Country.

December 1, 1992

Winter is here, and I'm back at work after a long Thanksgiving weekend. We had a wonderful time. I drove to Albany Wednesday night and had a delicious and entertaining holiday meal with Mom, M.R., Eddie, the boys and 200 Sisters of St. Joseph. Gary had volunteered to work at a shelter for the homeless where they served 1400 turkey dinners. I felt a bit guilty, but I know that I need to spend time with my family too. After the food and fun, I drove back to Canton. Friday we cooked our own Thanksgiving dinner, mostly to enjoy the leftovers, and spent the rest of the weekend pigging out, watching old movies, playing Scrabble and shopping for Christmas.

The quilt is here at St. Lawrence, 1400 panels of it anyway. Last night I went to see it. I have decided to design my own panel and asked a few friends whether or not they think it is a morbid or tasteless thing to do; they think not; so I will try it. I showed Gary some tentative designs, and he liked them.

Last week I had a visit from the man from the AIDS Task Force. His designated territory is Lewis and Jefferson counties, but he has been covering St. Lawrence County since the woman who had interviewed me in July quit. He told me that Jack, the guy I had for dinner a few times last spring, died in May. He got pneumonia and couldn't fight it off. This news upset me much more than I would have guessed, but I suppose I shouldn't be surprised. Although I have come to know many persons with HIV, I'm almost embarrassed at how few people I've known who have died.

Gary's last bloodwork came back with a big drop in the T-4 count—700 to 300 from July to November. He will have it taken again this week and will likely begin medicine if it is still that low. He is experiencing the same kick-in-the-gut reaction I had when I first began medication in July of 1990. I think no one can avoid the reaction; it always takes me a few days to recover from my visits to the doctor.

I got a letter from Jim yesterday; he told me that Maggie has only a few days to live, and that officials have named the new women's halfway house for her. I just stared at the note for a long time. Since the message was written on November 22, she may have died already. I will call Jim tonight to find out. I don't know what to write here. It amazes and saddens me that Maggie and I drifted apart in what I didn't know would be her last year of her life. She was one of the bright spots of my life when I lived in North Carolina. For two years, it was a rare day that we didn't at least talk with each other on the phone. When she found out about my infection, she cried and told me to "Come home" to North Carolina. She always said that she wasn't good at maintaining relationships after people moved on; so we arranged and had a meal specifically designed to punctuate our good-bye right before I left North Carolina three years ago. What an incredibly hard life, and what a remarkable woman! Dear Mags, there is nothing I can do now, but remember you, and that I will do well. I will love you always.

December 4, 1992

I called Jim when I got home from work the night before last. Maggie is alive, home and lucid when she is awake. Her pain-control medication is good at this point, and her brother is taking care of her. I called there but got the answering machine. I received calls from Kate, Mother and Ellen; so I was on the phone most of the evening. I finally told Jim about the HIV. I had been afraid about telling him, but he was great, and we had a wonderful and very funny talk.

I've been wrestling more than ever with the idea of moving. I'm feeling as if we are too remote, too far from the family, too far from good medical care—just too far—period. I'm afraid of getting sick and going to the hospital here. Though I understand that the hospital has improved to some degree in its handling of AIDS cases, it seems true also that there is a long way to go.

Jack, now dead, liked the care and treatment he received in Burlington. My doctor said the "locals" were better with his last patient, now dead also.

I just don't know what to do with myself. I guess I shouldn't feel hesitant to try for a different job elsewhere, but I do. The reason is mostly that I'll feel dishonest if I don't tell the new employers about the HIV, especially if I were to be sick soon thereafter. I really want not to go on disability before I need to, even though I could qualify now by virtue of my blood work. We could go to Albany where there is good medical care, or we could go to Ithaca, a nice community with so many things to offer, not so remote as Potsdam and, best of all, which counts Katy as one of its inhabitants. I remember dreaming of a return to N.C. For quite a while after the initial news of the infection, my desire to go back was so sharp that it hurt. I suppose my life is here now, somewhere in New York state.

I have decided to let it all simmer for now. The lease is up in July. If I still feel like this, maybe we'll make a change. Sometimes I just want to sell everything, load up the van and hit the road. I could see the country and maybe even find another planet to inhabit. Escape fantasies, I suppose!

December 18, 1992

It's the last full week before Christmas. It has been difficult getting into the holiday spirit this year. My shopping is halfway finished, and I don't know when I'll get to the rest of it. Tonight I'm going caroling with Julie, Barb, Dick, Cathy, Mike, Ginny and Steve. That should help instill some Christmas spirit into my veins. Gary has had a 400-point drop in his T-4 count since July; so he is beginning AZT. This is as depressing for him as it was for me. I had hoped that seeing me start medicine would ease the stress of it for him, but I think it doesn't work that way. For me, hearing that the virus is advancing is always a kick in the stomach. Why would that experience be any different for him?

Speaking of health or the lack of it, my liver enzymes are up, twice the normal count. They were good in September; so maybe the rise is due to the DDI.

I'd love to take a trip. If I get sick, so that I can't work, I have promised myself that I will take the van and drive around the country. The only obstacle might be mistaking what time is the best one to finish work. There is no question now. My body is my constant companion, and it isn't always friendly.

January 4, 1993

OK, I'll stop whining and admit that the holidays were fantastically wonderful. I have been so busy empathizing with clients about horrible holidays that I feel as though it is important, though perhaps unfashionable, to say I had a ball!

Gary and I went to Mother's house for Christmas Eve and Christmas night. The house had its usual Christmas-magic look, and Mary Rose, Katy, Charlie, Emma Rose, Max, Elizabeth, Eddie, Rosemary, Edward, Michael, Brian, Gary, and I rounded out Mom's guest list. The kids are terrific, and my gifts were a big hit. We recited our poems and sang our carols and, although nothing is ever the same without Ellen's renditions, it was a nearly perfect two days.

So, the holiday season is over once again, and there is so much for which I am grateful. I have made some New Year's resolutions. I will quit smoking. How many times before have I promised myself to do this? This promise will take effect later today when I will run out of my current pack of smokes. I have three cigarettes left. I will increase my exercise and my relaxation efforts, both of which have fallen by the wayside in recent months. I will decaf myself again. I have already cut way back from the ridiculously high levels of it I used to drink. My plan is to drink no more than three cups a day during the work week through January and then cut it out. We'll see.

January 7, 1993

Rudolf Nuryev died yesterday. In addition to this event, the medical community has changed the definition of the disease to include more conditions that affect HIV+ persons, especially women, and also, I believe, to include all those individuals with T-4 counts less than 200, even those who are asymptomatic. Thus, I am one of the 500,000+ Americans who officially have AIDS. Odd how disturbing it is to write this news even though the change is only definitional. I'm glad the virus doesn't know the new categories; it might obey symptomatically.

I am so sad about this disease today—not simply because I have it, but that it exists at all. I used to say that I liked who I was and who I was becoming. Since I really didn't know with any accuracy what episodes in my life shaped the results, there seemed to be little point in regrets. I know what I liked and what I didn't like, what was painful and what wasn't, but that's not the same thing as saying, "This was good for me; that wasn't." I always used to think I'd get busy with regrets as soon as I could figure out what parts of life weren't necessary to the person I had become.

I guess I still feel that way for everything except this virus. It has certainly taught me many things about myself, and that is good. However (and I hope I can say this without sounding grandiose), I was trying to learn those things before from easier teachers. And I'm sad because the world is really no different because of the disease. AIDS may have been a catalyst to the formation of an actual gay community where previously the term may have been primarily complimentary. AIDS may have increased everyone's awareness of a tolerance for diversity (though I'm unsure that even *that* is true), but what a cost for a catalyst—like using Clorox to cure irregularity. All those lives lost, talents squelched, tears shed, just to teach humans to be humans! I don't know. I guess if we didn't learn about compassion, acceptance, forgiveness and mercy from Jesus, we won't learn it from AIDS. Today I'd rather have everyone—gay and straight—still insensitive, still struggling but still alive.

January 15, 1993

I wonder whether or not the disease has begun for real with me? I have found a purplish-red mark on the underside of my right testicle. It looks like a blood blister. When I saw it, I broke out in a sweat and had to take a few deep breaths to calm down. I tried to remind myself that I'm only discovering evidence of a process that has been going on for nearly four years, to remember that I feel as good today as I felt yesterday before I found this mark. And, of course, maybe it isn't KS, though, frankly, it looks like every picture I've seen of it, and I can't imagine what else it might be—something benign maybe. To my surprise, I slept well last night, and I don't really have much to say about it today. I don't feel like calling the doctor and asking him to take a look. Part of the reason for this is that I think there is no effective treatment for it. A bigger part, however, is that I want not to hear my suspicion confirmed, especially if there is nothing to be done. Besides, I have heard that AIDS with Kaposi's Sarcoma has a slower progression than AIDS with pneumocystis. I guess that's good news.

January 28, 1993

I showed my growth to the doctor a week ago today, and basically he agreed with me that it looks like KS. He did some consultation work concerning what to do about it, including calling San Francisco. There's an AIDS hotline out there that he finds helpful. We're sticking with the plan to leave it alone. Although removal is certainly not a big deal, the only thing it would accomplish, apparently, is a definitive diagnosis of KS via a biopsy. The doctors still wouldn't have an effective treatment.

Excision, I guess, affects neither the likelihood of its recurring in that same spot nor its showing up elsewhere. They could do more radical treatment, i.e. some kind of chemo or radiation, but both the location of the lesion and the relative lack of success argue against those actions. It sounds as though the doctors resort to chemo and radiation only when the lesions are in some life-threatening place, and my location doesn't fit that bill; so we're letting the spot go for now, and I'll watch it. If the area begins to grow rapidly, we might do something else. I am at a choice point: I can submit myself to some aggressive treatments, or I can simply leave the lesion alone and hope it doesn't spread much farther. I tend to agree with the doctor that the latter choice is the way to go, but I want to investigate other possibilities. I have heard that the average life expectancy after discovering KS lesions is approximately eighteen months. As with everything else with this disease, it appears that there are enormous variabilities with an ever-growing number of long-term survivors even with KS. So, I make the next step in an endless chain of psychological adjustments and then get on with living (the dying stage of living, I guess).

On Monday night, I drove to Watertown to attend the HIV/AIDS support group meeting. It is a bit of a rush to get there by 7:00 p.m., especially if I stop to change my clothes, but it is doable. The meeting wasn't bad actually—nice people and a mix of HIV/AIDS and noninfected relatives. It was well attended, and I think I'll go again.

Ellen called me with Thomas' confirmation date—March 14. He is definitely choosing *John* for his confirmation name; I'm so happy about that. He's a wonderful and thoughtful kid, and taking *John* for me is a wonderful and thoughtful thing to do. I'm relieved that the confirmation is fairly soon as I am always these days when I make a promise to do something. I'm thinking that if I get new brakes in the van, I might even combine the trip to Kansas with some vacation time and drive down the Mississippi to New Orleans. My biggest concern is wondering whether or not it will be warm enough during that time of the year, so that the flowers from Natchez to Vicksburg will be in bloom. Probably a month later would be better; we'll see.

Clinton has been inaugurated. Among many claims that he is waffling about decisions and mishandling power, he is pushing to get the military to lift the ban on gays. People's reactions (especially those of the military brass) to the idea don't surprise me, but my own reaction to their ignorance is something I didn't count on. From officers in DC to enlisted men at bases around the country to an apparently furious middle America that has rung Congressional phones off the hook, the vituperativeness is stunning to me. Relatively few voices are even bothering to cloak their objections in a rational form, perhaps because none exists. Instead, they keep summoning up specters of predatory gay men in the barracks, showers and even foxholes, losing their minimal control and suddenly jumping all over unsuspecting straight soldiers.

I have always treasured diversity in my life. I have tried to value my friends simply because they are my friends regardless of the totally incidental aspects of what color they are and with whom they are involved in relationships. This attitude, however, has left me paranoid in a way I have never been. Maybe my friends, the straight ones, don't really like me, or if they do, maybe they are making one of those weird exceptions that humans are so good at (e.g. "He is not like other gay men."). This thinking is crazy, and I know it. What isn't crazy, however, is the always startling realization that there are so many persons who don't even know me but who would hate me simply because I am gay. There is even a good-sized element who would wish gay folks destroyed. Don't these people realize that we have enough physical, emotional and spiritual suffering of our own? I understand better individuals who go to live in gay ghettos in New York or San Francisco or someplace else just to forget feelings like these.

February 4, 1993

Nadine called me Monday to tell me that Maggie had died the night before. She had chosen to cease transfusions two weeks earlier when it became apparent that receiving the blood would only prolong an awful death. She became unconscious Thursday and died Sunday.

Dear Maggie, this is my good-bye to you. All week, my mind has returned to touching thoughts of our friendship. We had wonderful and funny times together in North Carolina when we were both healthy and working on becoming more so. I saw you struggle and prevail against horrendous abuse. I remember you were the person I called when I found out about the HIV, and you cried and asked me to "Come home." It is unbelievable to me that I sit here writing, and you are the one who is dead.

I now live at the northernmost part of the county in a place where winter's grip is secure for five months of the year. Nadine's news of your death comes at the coldest and most desolate point of the season.

June 11, 1993

This is surely the longest stretch between entries. I am making a retreat and brought this journal along with me partly to update it and partly to use the exercise of writing to focus my attention and energies.

My last entry was February 4 and was spurred on by Maggie's death. On the morning of February 13, our house burned down in a fire caused by my own improper disposing of a cigarette in the kitchen waste basket. I escaped wearing a bathrobe and slippers and, although the firefighters came quickly, the fire got into the rafters of the house, and saving the structure was out of the question. I called Barb in the middle of the night; she and Dick came over and got me, wrapped me in a blanket, took me to their house and put me to bed. I was up four hours later and went to see the house. Hard as I tried, there was nothing that could have prepared me for the sight of the house, still smoldering in the early winter light, covered with charred pieces of rafter. When I saw the inside, I cried. The place Gary and I had worked so hard on and were so proud of was gone. We had no place to live because of my own carelessness. I tried to tell myself to be grateful: Gary was in Albany and safe; the tenants are uninjured; I am fine; but I couldn't well up any truly grateful feelings. The hardest part was that I had killed the cat. And now, nearly six months later, I believe I am ready to write once again. I have come a long way in reconciling myself to all the losses except the loss of the cat. It's strange to me to think that I grew so fond of a cat. It's just that we took responsibility for her when we found her under the front porch, and she loved us back, even went into literal squirms of happiness when I came home from work. And while I do remember that we gave her a better and probably longer life that she would have had living wild, it is a hard thought that I ended her poor life.

I don't like to sound silly or indulgently self-hating, thus revealing what a sensitive man I am. I think I am just trying to say something about how that little life meant something to me. I'm sorry, Yods. I'm grateful also that it wasn't a person who died; it so easily could have been.

In March, Gary and I went to the AIDS unit at Albany Medical Center. The visit was partly to establish myself there, so that if I get sicker than the local hospital can handle, a better facility will at least have heard of me. I went also, however, because the KS lesion had spread rapidly to the point where I was often uncomfortable sitting because of the lesion rubbing against my pant legs. The doctors in Albany agreed with my local physician's opinion that the lesion should be treated.

In April, I began radiation treatments at Good Samaritan Hospital in Watertown, the nearest cancer treatment center to Potsdam. The treatment meant that every day I had to leave work early and drive two hours to get the five minutes of radiation, then drive two hours home. I did twenty sessions with a two-week hiatus in between because I got some severe, open and painful burns. I finally finished the radiation on M.R.'s birthday, May 20, and the treatment seems to have worked at least for now.

After the radiation had been completed, Gary and I finally took our long-planned vacation to New Orleans. We took the van and drove 4,000 miles in twelve days. We stopped in Ohio, Kentucky, Tennessee, DC, Virginia, North Carolina and Louisiana. We saw so many sights. It was exactly the trip I had had in mind for such a long time, and I'm thrilled that we chanced it.

June 12, 1993

I'm writing this while on retreat in the Adirondacks; I'm having a terribly difficult time with being here. Maybe it is just my usual couple of bad days after a doctor's appointment. I met with the doctor yesterday afternoon. Although the visit was uneventful, i.e., no change in the treatment plan, we did wind up talking about a living will and all that such a step involves. And even though I filled out mine over a year ago, I found the conversation disturbing—no, frightening—to be talking this over with my doctor. I guess that's what's wrong: I'm just flat out too scared of what's in store for me at some not-too-distant point in the future to be jolly up here on retreat. I hate saying this because it is also admitting (on paper even) a flaw in my otherwise flawless program for living with AIDS!

So I will pray: God, I think I know what is going to happen, and I want it not to happen. I'm afraid. Scared is OK, but it is now getting in the way of my life. Help me remember that I *have* enough within me to do this life, this death in a way of which I can be proud.

August 24, 1993

I haven't written in over two months. I don't feel so bad as I felt on the occasion of the last writing but am not embarrassed that I committed those feelings to paper, as I sometimes am when I reread my thoughts.

The summer is almost gone, and it has been a busy one. Gary and I started an HIV-support group here in Potsdam; we meet at our house on alternate Thursdays. We have had three meetings so far with seven HIV-infected persons. The meetings remind me that we have something to offer because the folks are amazingly honest although a bit unsophisticated about self-care and management.

Anyway, while I certainly do get tired, I feel a whole lot more engaged in my life and am a little more able to give a home in me to my struggles and pain as I am so easily able to do with my joys.

There are no major changes in my health, but there are some small ones. My skin is terribly dry which is sometimes very uncomfortable. I think the cancer (KS) is not coming back, but the one growth in my testicle that was the target of the radiation has, I think, turned to thick scar tissue that is often irritating.

I did have a bad night of fever a few weeks ago; in fact, my temperature reached 106 degrees before it broke that same evening. The doctor was on vacation, but his physician's assistant recommended a chest x-ray to look for pneumonia. The x-ray was scheduled for the next day, but I resisted because I was having no trouble breathing; also, my reasons were boiling down to childish denial. I wanted them not to find something that would require hospitalization. I know that this line of thinking is poor self-care, and I think I have resolved to be more attentive to the recommendations of the persons to whom I have entrusted myself. If I die, I surely hope it won't be because I am too much of a baby or a coward to seek the help I need.

August 25, 1993

I don't know what to write but figured it would do me good to scribble something anyhow. I find that sometimes the act itself primes the "feelings pump"— important for me since I'm not always so close to my feelings as perhaps I could and should be.

I don't think much about moving anymore. It used to be a constant debate in my mind. I couldn't figure out whether or not I wanted to stay here, especially when these healthy days come to a close. I felt trapped so much of the time. I think the house fire and resettling from Canton to Potsdam changed all that. There is nothing like a forced move to cure the desire for an elective one. In addition, I have come to recognize that no matter where I go, I would go there in this HIV-infected body, and there is no place to hide from that reality.

So I have refocused for now on the goodness of my area: my job, our new home and my relationship with Gary. And the refocusing has worked.

I still haven't talked about my AIDS with anyone in the family but Katy. Before her visit here in July, M.R. sent me a card, and I know her message was an overture or an invitation to talk during her visit. She and Sister Pat came for just an overnight, and I didn't feel like ruining their trip with my news. That's a funny statement because if M.R. knows, then it probably ruined her trip that I didn't tell her. One thing I do know: it is up to me because even if they get suspicious or are so already, my family will try to respect my timing. It is funny to think of my family and how they will react; there is no question in my mind about their love for me lasting forever; I'm just not ready to have them camped out on my doorstep. And as wonderful as they are and as understanding as they will be, it will still be so difficult. I read somewhere recently that gay people are the only minority who come from families who are not members of that minority, and that is a suffering all by itself.

August 27, 1993

I'm reading David McCullough's biography of Harry Truman, and I am full of admiration for the author and the subject. His description of middle America at the end of the nineteenth century does, indeed, make it seem as if we have lost something of our national character: traits like self-reliance, accountability, personal integrity, hard work. The author by no means idealizes the period in the funny way that Ronald Reagan and Dan Quayle idealized it. In fact, in some respects, notably our awareness of and sensitivity to diversity, we have come quite a long way. (Harry Truman regularly wrote letters to Bess that today would be considered blatantly and unforgivably racist.) Anyhow, it's a wonderful portrait of a man and the times that shaped him.

September 1, 1993

Today is the first day of my birthday month. It feels as if the end of summer has come in spite of the fact that it is very hot. Perhaps it's the coolness of the night; no doubt it's the wonderful return of the college students. Although I lose the easy parking at work, it is always exciting for me to see the kids come back; everything about them seems fresh and new and happy.

It's quite good news on the health front. I had a doctor's appointment here in Potsdam on Friday and one at the cancer center in Watertown on Monday. I have gained five pounds and am back to 180—a good weight for my 6' 2" frame. Dr. Joe in Watertown thinks my KS lesion looks better and gave me a six-month follow-up appointment; anyone who gives me a six-month follow-up these days becomes my best friend automatically!

I had a good weekend; my spirit was buoyed tremendously by the medical news. I called Kate Friday night and spent two hours talking with her, mostly laughing with her at lots of hilarious statements and situations.

Right now I am actually thinking of beginning my Christmas shopping. Whether or not this is an impulse I'll fight off, I don't know, but it's weird that, by summer's end, I'm starting to make plans for Christmas. Somehow I must believe that if I'm ready for Christmas, I'll be sure to be alive at Christmas.

Labor Day weekend is coming up, and I'd like to do something. Possibilities include the State Fair in Syracuse, the ocean somewhere, a camping trip or to Latham to see Mary Rose. Mom is at camp with the widows and orphans; they have been going for Labor Day for so long now that it is a real tradition. Mom's friends are the kind of support group that any psychologist would recommend.

September 3, 1993

This is the first day of the long weekend, and it is pouring. I still haven't figured out vacation plans, and the weather isn't helping. I have an itch to buy a new computer and a camcorder, but I'm not sure how practical an idea that is. Essentially, they are toys, and I don't know how much we need either one. I'd use the camcorder to tape our trips and holiday gatherings and to record some messages for my family for the future. I'd use the computer definitely more as a toy than for anything else. I've considered getting a decent printer and word-processing program to use when I am no longer able to work.

There is always the annoying conflict in my mind: *Will I be well enough long enough to justify these expenses?* and *Why not spend it all?* Maybe we'll have a garage sale quickly before the summer officially ends; I wouldn't feel guilty spending any of that money on new toys.

September 13, 1993

It's really fall, and the weather is still warm, but we are getting the wind that seems so peculiar to September. Some of the trees—I think the old and the sick ones—are already giving up their green to the evening snap of chill. I like the way that trees go out in a glorious blaze of color as if they not only are *accepting* the changes of the season but also are *celebrating* their surrender to those changes.

Saturday night Gary and I watched the HBO premiere of *And the Band Played On*. The producers did a good job of dramatizing the book, I thought, but the anger that I remember as one of the book's chief virtues seemed watered down to me in the film. Strangely, some of the most inherently dramatic aspects of the story seemed overlooked in the movie. This is quibbling, though; the flick was well made and powerful even on its own.

Also, the program prompted one of the few talks Gary and I have had lately about our situation. We took a long walk after the movie was over and discussed quietly what this disease is doing to us individually and as a couple. I suppose it is a coping style for us that we don't spend a great deal of time talking about the virus, but it felt good to talk Saturday night. The conversation reminded me of how difficult and how rarely accomplished it is that I am able to reach outside myself and touch another person soul to soul. I think God was in the effort Saturday.

I spoke about my fears. I have heard persons say that they aren't afraid of death; they're afraid of dying. I'm afraid of the whole deal. The movie portrayed several AIDS patients who were covered with KS lesions all over their faces. At least mine don't show yet. I find myself bargaining with God again, this time asking to be spared of cytomegalovirus retinitis and toxoplasmosis. Just maybe I can cope if I still have my sight and my mind. I don't want disfigurement; I don't want pain; I don't want to find out whether or not I can suffer and die with some semblance of dignity.

I'm in some pain from the lesions, especially from two dime-shaped sores that are proving slow to heal. I'm washing with an antibiotic soap, am using Vitamin E which is supposed to help skin quality after radiation and am taking Tylenol #3 for the pain, but it is getting more and more difficult to walk.

My skin is generally worse off these days. It is so dry that it itches, and I have to be careful because just a little absent-minded scratching opens up the skin. I read about an alternative treatment in the AIDS newsletter called DNCB, a substance one paints on to provoke a cell-mediated response resembling poison ivy or poison oak. Some scientists think it is useful in boosting T cells; it is used also to treat warts in children. I've contacted the address in San Francisco for a price list.

I talked with M.R. and Mom this weekend. We are all going to meet at Katy and Charlie's this weekend to celebrate Max's and my birthdays. He will be 3; I'll be 36. It will be fun and, best of all, I've made it to another year.

September 27, 1993

A good deal has happened since I last wrote. On September 17, my boss and good friend, Sandy, died of cancer at age 47. She had been off work for only a week, and although most of us were aware that she was ill again, we were shocked at the suddenness of her death. Sandy was wonderful to me—always sensible and very kind. She was private about whatever fear and pain she faced, mentioning them only when she thought the disclosure might be helpful to someone else. She was so supportive of me when I was having the radiation treatments last spring, allowing me the time I needed from my work schedule to drive every day to Watertown. I think her behavior, in many ways, set the tone for our relationships with one another here at the clinic. In addition, she was, for me, a model of how to face murderous adversity. Whatever I am called on to do, to suffer, I hope to be able to do half as well as Sandy did. We are quite devastated here at the clinic.

Before Sandy's wake and funeral, I had time to drive to Ithaca, as planned, to celebrate birthdays (Emma Rose's, Max's and mine) with Mom, Mary Rose, Katy, Charlie, Emma Rose, Max and Elizabeth. We had a marvelously fun and funny time, and the kids went crazy opening presents. I didn't do too badly myself. So, now I am 36.

Gary and I went to Ogdensburg Monday to see Jim, one of the members of our support group, who is hospitalized with his sixth bout with pneumonia. He looks OK, but breathing exhausts him. I just got off the phone with him this morning, and he tells me he may be discharged this week; if so, he will be in a wheelchair with oxygen. Although he is very sick, his spirits are quite good. I think he sounds more hopeful about living than he is frightened of dying. We will move the group meeting to his place, so that he doesn't have to travel to make it. It seems to mean a lot to him that we get together.

This past weekend, I got sort of overwhelmed by everything and just wanted to be by myself. I seem to need more time and space these days than I used to need, and it disturbs me a bit that I want to talk with fewer and fewer persons. I wonder if this feeling has something to do with drawing away to die. However, since I am still working, and associating with people is a requisite, I need to make a point of scheduling one or two social events each week simply to keep myself engaged.

Anyway, social engagement is not what I wanted this weekend; so with Gary's understanding, I took the van and drove by myself to Meacham Lake to the canoe launch. The leaves are changing now, and nothing smells so good in the autumn air as the wood smoke from the maple fire I built. I sat by my fire watching the lake and, to my delight, was observed, in turn, by a small family of raccoons who kept peeking out at me from the tree behind which they were hiding. I read two books by the light of the van and later, when it started to rain, I slept peacefully to the sound of the rain on the van's steel roof. At one point I remember noticing how much the inside of the van looks like a coffin with its metal hull and its padded walls and ceiling. I laughed out loud thinking maybe I could be buried in the van itself on a truly extended camping trip.

The brief getaway did what I had hoped it would do, and I felt better able to come back to my life with arms out and eyes open.

I read a poem recently that I think is by Stanley Kunitz, whom I once heard speak at a conference at Notre Dame. I may be paraphrasing here, but the poem goes something like this:

> *In these murderous times,*
> *The heart breaks and breaks and breaks,*
> *And lives by breaking.*

October 1, 1993

I made an appointment to see the doctor about a month sooner than my next scheduled visit. I wanted to talk with him about my skin. I am incredibly dry everywhere which means I am also very uncomfortable itching; this is something that will only get worse with the onset of winter. Basically, it seems that I am doing everything I can do. In addition, I have a minor fungal infection on my foot and got some Nizoral cream for that.

Besides all of those complaints, I asked the doctor to look at the KS lesions on my upper leg. The sores there still haven't healed, and I have had them about six weeks. I have been taking Tylenol #3 and spraying with a topical anesthetic. Some days they are very painful, especially when the T #3 wears off. The doctor recommended that I get off the sprays and use a particular antibiotic/anesthetic cream; we agreed that I could begin a stronger pain killer; so I started with Percocet. At the start of the discussion, I was hesitant about using what seemed like such a strong drug, but the doctor made a good point that the pain can erode my general ability to cope, and that's true. Sometimes at the end of a workday, I feel overwhelmed, and it is always when the pain has worn me down. This can't be good for my overall well-being.

As far as the causes of the problems, the doctor speculated it was either a change in skin quality because of the radiation or possibly more of the KS. What is true is that I am getting more spots on the inside of my upper thigh. These marks are the big reason for my getting an earlier appointment. We talked about more radiation and possibly systemic chemotherapy, but I don't feel informed or equipped to make the choice of treatment at this point. The radiation can shrink, even kill the lesions upon which it is aimed but doesn't reduce the chances of recurrence in that spot or elsewhere. Apparently the chemo can do a better job, but the accompanying sickness is awful. My quality of life might be better if I simply let the lesions do whatever they do.

We decided on a consult with a dermatologist acquainted with AIDS and KS. My choices are Burlington (University of Vermont), Syracuse, Albany Medical Center or Rochester. I have been to the first three at various times. I don't care for Syracuse, and neither does my local doctor. Burlington, though a regional AIDS center for Northern New England, is still rather small. I had made a contact with Albany Med earlier this year and very much liked the doctor there; it was she who helped me decide to radiate the KS last March.

Since lunch when I wrote the above paragraph, I have heard from my doctor here who spoke with the specialist at Albany Medical Center. She doubts that the sores on my thigh are KS lesions but rather slow-healing ulcers from radiation burns. She recommends that we freeze the spots on my leg if they continue to spread quickly. In addition, she gave us the name of her favorite dermatologist (in Poughkeepsie) to keep in reserve; so we will try freezing these bad boys at the end of the month.

We have a new member of the support group who is quite involved with hospice at this point. He has KS lesions all over his body and is wheelchair bound because of the edema in his legs. He understands that this swelling and inability to stand is the result of KS in his groin which blocks off the lymph glands and thus the circulation. Gary and I spoke with him at separate times via the phone. He wants to come to the meetings but needs a ride. I will visit him soon because I think he is quite lonely up here. The thought of the visit is frightening because my doctor warned me that it may be upsetting, something about which I had already thought. I dread the disfigurement this man evidently has and which may very well be in my own future. This dread, however, feels like astonishing selfishness and quite beside the point.

I have ordered, received and started some new supplements and alternative choices from the buyer's club in San Francisco, including the DNCB. I painted my arm with the latter last night and now have a nice little rash; so I guess I'm reacting. Other new additions include NAC, Vitamins C, E, B Complex, Beta Carotene, Zinc and Selenium; these are supplemental to my prophylaxes, AZT and DDI. I must have a cast-iron stomach for which I guess I am grateful.

I have decided to drive to Albany tomorrow to talk with Mary Rose. I think she knows and is respecting my timing but maybe not. Somehow the weight against having the conversation shifted yesterday. I can't go on without my family's knowing. Telling M.R. will give Katy someone with whom to talk and may help me figure out how to tell Mom and everyone else. This is a horrible mission I am on.

October 4, 1993

I am still stunned. Mary Rose *did* know—not suspected but *knew*. I went down to the Provincial House Saturday, and we sat in her office all day and talked. When I began the conversation, my mind was spinning and my hands were visibly shaking, a fact I attributed to too much coffee. After the pause in the dialogue that I knew would come, a pause I had both prayed for and dreaded, I said, "M.R., this visit isn't completely impulsive." She had a dear smile on her face that allowed me to keep looking at her, something I didn't know if I would be able to do. She said very simply, "I know." I couldn't believe we were on the same track because not only was she calm but also quite visibly at peace. Her love for me was reflected in her eyes, and I said, "Are we talking about the same thing?" Mary Rose said, "Yes, your health, J.R.; I wanted you to come, and I didn't want you to come. When you didn't come, I could, at least for a while, convince myself you were healthy. I know you have AIDS; I've never been sadder; and I've never loved you more."

As our conversation continued, Mary Rose told me that she had seen my AZT bottle six months ago when she moved my suitcase from her bed on the sunporch at my mother's to the bed where I would be sleeping. She recognized the name "Retrovir" immediately because prior to her beginning an experimental treatment in New York City for a bad foot ulcer, M.R. had to have an AIDS test because the treatment involved reusing part of her own blood in some form. When she asked the doctor what he would do if the test were positive (She had had numerous blood transfusions.), he said they would probably use a medicine called "Retrovir." When M.R. saw my AZT, she said her heart sank, and she began hoping that maybe I was taking the medicine as a preventive measure, although her research didn't support such a practice.

When Gary would say to me that he was sure M.R. knew about my situation but was respecting my choice not to share the information, I always said he was wrong—that if she knew she would be camped out at my doorstep. Fully cognizant of her love for me, I misjudged her strength and her respect for my own privacy. We talked all day and into the early hours of the morning, breaking to pick up Sister Pat who had played at a wedding that evening. Pat played a beautiful piece for me on the St. James organ, and I had a chance to talk with her, too, about myself and AIDS. Her tremendously warm, sincere and loving hug touched me deeply and assured me that Mary Rose would have the support she would need when I left.

Dearest M.R., I feel that one of my heaviest burdens has been lifted. Your love has been one of the constants in my life, and your own suffering has given me a much needed model. I love you, biggest sister.

October 12, 1993

I didn't finish the entry for October 4. Last night, M.R. called to tell me that she had talked with Ellen this weekend when Ellen came to Utica for a visit. We had agreed that this was a good idea because it would be too difficult for Ellen to learn of the news through a phone call to Kansas City. I had asked Mary Rose not to tell Mother or Eddie because I would like to do that myself. M.R. said that she and Ellen talked and cried for many hours, and that Ellen was OK, or as M.R. put it, "As OK as heartbroken can be."

For reasons I don't really understand, I started to cry when I was talking with Mary Rose. She was wonderful and calm with me, and I assured her that my tears on the phone were unusual—that I'm not normally such a mess—which is true. I had talked to Kate on Friday night, and she wound up sobbing during that conversation. If I feel guilty about anything connected with having AIDS, it is about the pain I am causing my family, all of whom have treated me my entire life as if I were something very special. Even now, their love and concern for me shine through their grief and pain, and I feel so terribly sad and so incredibly grateful.

Now I can talk more freely about the whole situation. It has been a couple of months since the sores in my groin opened up, and I am more than a little worn down by them. I am taking Percocet tablets and trying to avoid the topical anesthetics because, while they work, they keep the area too moist to heal properly.

In addition, the KS lesions are spreading. They are now on my upper right thigh, emerging in about a two-inch circle. After talking with the doctor in Albany, my doctor here told me we could try freezing them in his office, or I could go back to Watertown for more radiation. I have ordered some shark cartilage which some people believe is helpful in battling cancer. I don't know how convincing the written material is, but I have nothing to lose at this point.

I have just had a three-day weekend and am still tired. I don't feel great today, and I am considering leaving work after my 1:00 p.m. appointment. Sometimes I think it is time to quit work, but more often I think I should stay for as long as I can do the job effectively.

I'm trying to pray, but today I looked at the lesions and am reminded of William Blake's line to the Tyger: *"Did He who made the Lamb make thee?"*

October 25, 1993

It's a beautiful fall day. We have had an unusually windy season, and all the leaves are down, but right now the sky is clear and the grass, where it isn't covered, is still green. It's the kind of day I associate with L.L. Bean outerwear.

Mother came for a visit yesterday. She stayed overnight with us and left this morning shortly after I went to work. I think she had a good time; I know I did. In any case, I was thrilled that she came. Gary and I cleaned the house like crazy, and I made a Sunday dinner which came out just right. After dinner, the three of us just visited. Besides the fact that I have loved Mother longer and deeper than anyone else in my life, she has always been my very favorite person just to sit and talk with. I was struck again by that last night and this morning at breakfast. Gary enjoys her greatly, and I think she was pleased with the house. I need to talk with Mother soon about my HIV status, but I keep thinking, "Just one more good time." Besides, I can't imagine her driving home alone with that information. Then I remember reading recently Dan Berrigan's description of his mother; in the beginning of the piece he says that she "might safely have been entrusted with the fate of the world." I think Mrs. Berrigan and my mother might be related. Mom will make it through with me.

I went to see the local dermatologist about the new lesions on my upper inside thigh. He took a culture, prescribed a lidocaine gel for the pain and told me to get off the over-the-counter anesthetic I had been using. In addition, he suggested that, since I had had good results with the previous radiation, I should have the new lesions radiated as soon as possible. I have an appointment in Watertown the day after tomorrow and will probably begin treatments immediately. My hope, of course, is that the treatments will work as well as they worked before; I got the shark cartilage which I will use in conjunction with the radiation. A secondary hope, one I think is reasonable, is that if I burn, maybe it won't hurt so much because of the previous scarring. I was going to enroll in an experimental chemo program for KS patients in New York City but decided to hold off until the radiation is complete. The New York program would require sixteen weekly visits. A bigger concern or at least the backdrop to all this is the consideration of whether or not the antiretrovirals I am on (AZT and DDI) are still working for me; I keep getting new lesions now on an almost daily basis.

It was a good weekend. For most of the past few weeks, I would get home from work, change into sweat pants and watch TV; I was hurting and very tired. It felt so good to run errands on Saturday and visit with Mom on Sunday. In fact, today I feel as restored as if I had been on a vacation.

Gary and I went to visit Rick early Saturday morning. (Rick is the new member of our group whom I hadn't yet met.) Gary had been over several times during the week to see him while I was at work. We brought him some of the most beautiful roses I have ever seen and from our own garden at that. Rick was in a much worse condition than I had expected he would be. The doctor was a bit concerned about my seeing him, partly because he is riddled with infections—herpes sores, CMV and who knows what else—and also because he is covered with KS lesions. One of his legs looks like a huge purple sausage, and the rest of him—chest, face and body—is spotted liberally with lesions big and small.

I am very happy I went. I think of persons in geographic areas where AIDS has hit with greater impact, those who have watched friend after friend wind up looking like Rick, many knowing a similar outcome was waiting for them. How could I not go? In addition, Rick had left most of his support system in Dallas and had come up here to die. He is very nice and very gentle.

I hadn't counted on what the visit would do *for* me; I was worried (and selfishly so) only about what it might do *to* me. I can't explain my feelings well here, but I found Rick to be quite beautiful. He was proof to me that there is something that animates our being even when horrible things are happening to our bodies. I think Rick must have had great openness to that grace. He did me a greater service than a bunch of flowers, no matter how beautiful, and a visit from me could do for him.

December 15, 1993

Another long period between entries. So much has happened. I began radiation treatments at the end of October for the lesions on the inside of my right thigh; the routine involved daily trips to Watertown, about two hours each way. They couldn't treat me at the end of the day as they had done in the spring. I asked for an early time, so that I could work at least part of the day. It is difficult and tiring to get the treatments, then travel and go to work, but it is the best we could figure. I have been trying to minimize the impact of my absence on clients and think I have done a fair job of it, but the effort means that my afternoons are jammed with every appointment slot filled. I don't know how much longer I can keep up the schedule.

I got through the fifteen treatments on my leg, finishing

shortly before Thanksgiving. As I had hoped, there were no burns painful or significant enough to halt the treatments. Unfortunately, over the Thanksgiving weekend while we were in Utica visiting Mom, the area began to hurt; it turned out that I had a staph infection which looked to me like a strep throat with lots of little blisters that tended to break open and stick to whatever I was wearing. This infection, combined with the long-standing ulcers on my thigh, has made pain management the biggest part of my program these past few weeks. I think, however, that both conditions are resolving themselves finally. My leg is drying up, and the blistered skin is peeling off. I can hardly remember the days when a normal scab would form on a sore, dry up and fall off, leaving little or no evidence of injury.

Unfortunately, there were further developments. In the course of the radiation on my leg, I discovered three more areas of developing lesions on the left side of my thigh and groin; so now the new lesions have to be treated, and nearly two months after I began, Watertown is still a part of my life. I have eight treatments remaining on one of the areas and nine each on the other two. I am currently on hold for a week, but I can see that the folks who do the radiation in Watertown are getting discouraged with my lack of results. The new areas simply keep coming faster than we can radiate them. Given the condition of my skin from the previous treatments, I think they are reluctant (as I am) to continue.

This development is disturbing to me and very scary. I really feel that I'm not ready yet to say simply, "The treatment isn't worth it; let the lesions go." But I am also sick of driving, sick of burns, sick of infections and sick of pain in the radiated area. I'm going to try to finish this session, and then I will explore any remaining options with the KS specialist recommended to me earlier. I know that chemo is one option, but does it ever really work for KS? And do I want to be that sick at this time of my life with no real payoff? My lesions are now extremely angry looking, and the deep radiation wound is raw, weeping and refusing to heal. In truth, my whole leg is red, swollen and suppurating continuously. I drove back to Watertown yesterday thinking that maybe it is getting near the time when I need to focus more on quality of life than on pursuing treatments that may extend it for awhile but leave me in pain the whole time.

The week following Thanksgiving required a break from the radiation because I got sick. On November 25, I started running a fever, which quickly rose to 105 degrees. I went to bed, hoping the fever would break during the night as it had done in the past; it did break but dropped only to 101-102 degrees and then rose again. I saw the doctor Monday night, and he thought he heard a bit of pneumonia in my right lung. He was right according to the x-rays and workup I had at the hospital, but it was a light case and not PCP. AIDS is definitely a good source for bad news/good news jokes. The pneumonia was not a big problem as far as breathing goes, and my oxygen level stayed high. I had a cough but no more than I had had for a time. I wasn't hospitalized but stayed out of work for a few days. The fever was gone by Tuesday, allowing me the luxury to return to trying to ignore my pain once again.

The timing of all these complications wasn't the best. Gary had to go to North Carolina to cater his sister's wedding, was leaving Friday morning and was planning to be gone through the following week. Originally, I was going along to help him work, but the radiation screwed that up; so I was going to go as company and help with sit-down activities such as making phone calls to food and rental companies. The pneumonia ruined that plan, and we ended up deciding he would go alone. I kept the vacation time I had already blocked out, went to Watertown in the mornings and came home to rest in the afternoons. I think the rest and quiet did me good.

Gary's catering at the wedding came off beautifully, and he is very proud of the results. I worry about him every day because his counts are in the low 200s. He hasn't felt good but has no specific complaints and thinks he is only overtired from the reception. We joke at night about being two little old men trying to take care of ourselves and each other. If the tables turn and his acute needs become greater than mine, I hope I can be as good and patient with him as he has been with me.

December 16, 1993

There is more than I had time to write about yesterday. Rick died on December 3, the same day Gary left for North Carolina and the end of the week of my mild pneumonia. Rick had a terribly painful week previous to his death; so how sad can one be about his move to a more peaceful and pain-free place? I so admired his unforced sincerity and gentleness, and I wish his spirit well. I went to his wake Saturday by myself since Gary had already left for North Carolina. The casket was open and Rick looked very tranquil. His mother had placed his birth bracelet on his wrist; that gesture made me cry thinking of all the mothers who have seen their children grow up only to die of this disease. I keep reminding myself that God is as present in the sad things of life as in the happy ones; it's a hard reminder.

The most important part of this entry is that December 3 was also the weekend that Mary Rose had gone to Utica to talk with Mother about my having AIDS. After Thanksgiving, the time I told her I would tell Mom (and then couldn't), she called me to say that my symptoms were now very obvious, that Mom kept asking if anything were wrong and that I was not being fair. She understood that I wanted to tell Mother myself but noticed that I froze whenever I tried to do it. She offered to tell Mom for me, and I was touched and relieved. For quite a long time, I felt as if I could talk to Mom about having the disease if I could only get out the initial phrase, "Mom, I have AIDS." I can't and M.R.

is right; the time has come. I fought as hard as I could, but the virus fought harder.

Mary Rose went on Saturday and stayed with Mother until Wednesday. How can I ever describe my love for my sister or the debt I owe her for taking on what I know was the hardest task of her life? After she had told Mom, M.R. went up to tell Eddie and said he was terribly shocked and immediately supportive. I wonder at the limitless capacity of my family to make love real through their actions.

Mother was wonderful. That remarkable woman who gave me this terrific life called and said simply, "I'm so sorry, dear, and I'm so sad. I'll do whatever I can. I love you, and I'll call you later." I knew she was going to cry and cry, and the heartbreak from which I had wanted so long to spare her had finally arrived, but at that moment, my mother said just enough to make me realize my worries were over. Later that night, Mom called back, and we had a long, long talk. During the day, she had gone to tell a few of her closest friends. I so admire her healthy instinct to share her sorrows as well as her joys, especially this sorrow which so many have kept a secret. I feel a peace I haven't experienced for years. *The singing bird has come.*

I have thought often before now and have perhaps written in these pages that I am humbled to have been part of this family and, particularly, the son of this woman. It is she who taught me that my life is a gift, my happiness a choice, and that always, no matter what, love heals. To you who have loved me longer and harder than anyone, dear Mother, to you, all my love.

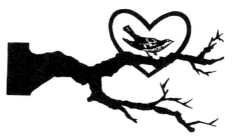

EPILOGUE

Dick's Death—Choice, Loss and Gift

Dick died of complications from the AIDS virus on May 6, 1994—four years, seven months and eight days after his initial diagnosis and five and one-half months after his last journal entry. I believe he wrote most often during times of struggle, conversing with himself about his inner peacemaking. When all of his family and friends had learned of his health status, his monologues could become dialogues, and he no longer needed to write.

Those last months of Dick's life were a release from his inability to communicate for such a long time. It wasn't perfect. He had already experienced, to some degree, all of Elisabeth Kübler-Ross' stages of death—denial, anger, bargaining with God, depression, acceptance. Sometimes, one stage replaced another; at other times, more than one stage existed side by side. However, we hadn't even begun. Thus, time gave us opportunities to express our anger, to cry out our grief, to articulate our fears, to move—slowly we hoped— toward our separation from Dick. Those months gave us a little time to pull together to face the inevitable.

In his journal, Dick spoke of how easy it was for him to talk about having AIDS once the news was widespread—and talk he did. In many ways, the ordinary remained ordinary; joys were still joys; agonies were still agonies. In many other ways, however, we were all with Dick and Gary on a seesaw, going back and forth, up and down, between fear of death and promise of eternity.

Dick tried to think of death as a mere biological event, as a natural experience of moving on, and he described to us his journey of coming to grips with the mystery of his own life—his feelings of resentment, fear, guilt, shame. During one conversation, Dick said that when he finally admitted to himself in his late twenties that he was, indeed, a gay man, much of his inner struggling was over, and he felt a new sense of freedom. He remembered that feeling when he got sick, and the memory helped him. Just as Dick longed to be free of the burden of hiding his disease, so did he eventually long to be free from the limits of the earth as we know it. When he was planning his funeral with Pat Houlihan, CSJ, a family friend, Dick described how he longed for completion, how he desired to be radically free beyond the limits of time and space, suffering and pain. As Dick became sicker and sicker, he became more and more convinced also that death was the **only** way to reach the freedom of what was beyond that step.

In so many ways, Dick actively experienced death, making choices all along the way. That is not to say that denial, anger and depression stayed away. He felt it especially ironic that he had to come to accept his dying so soon after he had come to accept himself as a gay man. He was filled with questions, and so were we. Nor is it to say that he gave up. Until a month before his death, Dick left room for the possibility of a cure, for the discovery of a new therapy. He continued treatments at Albany Medical Center and was very grateful that his physician included him in all decisions and allowed him some hope. When that same doctor finally said, "Let's stop the treatments; you have suffered enough, and you have done it all so well," Dick felt peace and acceptance—even pride at having his struggles so recognized. He left the medical center that day, ready to meet the challenges of his last few weeks. When I watched Dick walk down the corridor that afternoon—on his own but with extreme difficulty—I saw in him a tremendous testimony to the strength and grit of the human spirit.

One of Dick's favorite topics of conversation with me during those weeks was what heaven would be like. The image of a place where little cherubim and seraphim danced around was not exciting to Dick, nor was a place of *eternal rest*. What he liked to imagine was a state of complete freedom, of perfect relationships, of unbounded compassion and forgiveness. He hoped deeply and believed nearly as much that he would be able to recognize and communicate with loved ones who had predeceased him, especially my father and my grandmother.

In a sense, the way Dick chose to die set his family and friends free to mourn him, not with remorse or guilt, but with gratitude. So many of Dick's fears were spared. An avid reader throughout his life and an old-movie aficionado, Dick knew that those two hobbies would help to assuage his pain and pass time; so he hoped to keep his mind and his eyesight intact. While he suffered months of agonizing pain from bone-deep Kaposi's sarcoma lesions, Dick had no CMU retinitis, no pneumocystic pneumonia and no toxoplasmosis; his sight and his mind were with him until the moment he left this world. In fact, the night before he died, Dick played *Jeopardy* with Barb, Gary, Ellen and my mother—and he won!

We who loved Dick have lived continuously with the heartache and grief of his suffering, yet not without memories of an amazing surrender and pride in a tremendous triumph of integrity. Pain gave Dick an unusual openness to grace. He knew that within his own heart was the wisdom to choose the way to go. And while he saw callousness and indifference in the world around him and experienced his own feelings of anger, frustration and impotence, Dick chose to focus on kindness, compassion and trust. In so doing, he helped all of us to contemplate more deeply the mystery at the very heart of life.

Dick's journey into his own humanity made him humble and dependent. At the same time, it enabled him to touch the core of his divinity, that essence that can come only from a Higher Being. He struggled to see God's transcendent life, and he emerged victorious. When he came to the doors of death and was stripped literally to his essence, it was awesome to see what was there. Beyond his love for family and friends, beyond his successful career, beyond his many gifts of nature and grace was a drive toward what is mysterious and incomprehensible.

If a prescient angel or a rising star could take Dick our thoughts this day, he would know that we have been awed by his focus, moved by his courage, inspired by his faith.

At Dick's funeral, Monsignor H. Charles Sewall described him by using Marc Antony's final tribute to Brutus in Shakespeare's **Julius Caesar:**

> *His life was gentle, and the elements*
> *So mix'd in him that Nature might stand up*
> *and say to all the world, "This was a man!"*

And this man reached his final freedom, hard won and well deserved. Our brother was noble, indeed, in life and in death.

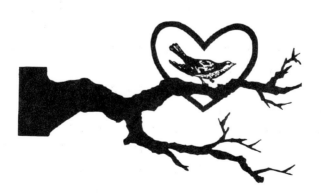

AFTERWARD

Washington, DC—The Quilt, 1996

During the Columbus Day weekend last year, Eddie, Ellen, Katy and I traveled from Utica, Kansas City, Ithaca and Albany to Washington, DC, to present a panel in memory of Dick to the NAMES Project's National AIDS Quilt. There we met Gary who had moved to the South after Dick's death to be near his family. (Gary continues to hold his own and is taking one of the new drug-combination treatments for AIDS.)

The story of our panel presentation began in 1994. When Dick was near death, he sketched his own design for the piece "in case we ever felt inclined to present one." We talked about the idea several times during our moments of shared grieving and made tentative plans for implementing Dick's design. Last summer, Ellen, with the help of friends in Kansas City, completed the beautiful panel which centered on a bouquet of five different-colored sweetheart roses, four in the vase with Dick's having fallen out of the bouquet onto the table. We passed from house to house Ellen's work of art, and we all wrote a message and signed our names to the panel.

During the weekend in Washington, nearly a million individuals viewed the quilt which stretched along the National Mall from the Washington Monument to the Capitol. As far as we could see, there were colorful, fabric tributes, and we knew that those remembrances could only hint at the lives behind them. There were panels for such persons as: Arthur Ashe, tennis player; Michael Callen, singer; Michael Bennett, choreographer; Perry Ellis, fashion designer; Michel Foucault, philosopher; Rock Hudson, actor; Stewart McKinley, U.S. congressman; Keith

Haring, artist; Liberace, pianist; Rudolf Nureyev, dancer; Dr. Tom Waddell, olympian; there were panels for teachers, lawyers, chefs, priests, rabbis, policemen, beauticians, children, parents, grandparents and now, a panel for Dick Noonan, son, brother, uncle, friend.

Presenting Dick's panel was an opportunity to tell his story once again. Along with the piece, we gave to the NAMES Project Archives a letter, a written description of the panel, a photo of Dick and a copy of his obituary, all of which spoke to our experience with AIDS, and we felt that, in some way, we were passing on Dick's legacy to future generations.

AIDS came on Dick and on us with unexpected and cruel abandon. It forced us to look, together with our beloved brother, at the frailty of our beings and at the reality of death, and it was the most difficult thing we have ever done. Like most of our culture, we didn't enjoy talking about death, but we no longer had the luxury of avoiding it.

We realize that Dick's suffering and his death have changed our whole world, and each of us has passed through times when we feared the grief would be so unbearable that we might get lost on the journey. We didn't get lost, however, and I think we realize now that it is exactly the grieving that has held us together. When I looked at all of my siblings in Washington and thought of my mother who was praying for us at home, I realized that, in many ways, the AIDS experience has brought out the best in us, and it was right that we were taking our mourning one step further to grieve with the whole human family. In our shared vulnerability, God was powerfully present, and in that large crowd of persons who were grieving and giving thanks at the same time, it was evident that God, indeed, is Love.

We could not possibly have been prepared for the effect that seeing the entire quilt would have on us; the glimpse of the lives behind the statistics and the magnitude of the epidemic are simply overpowering. Sunday, we returned to the quilt, took off our shoes, crawled out to the panel, touched it and said *good-bye* to Dick one more time.

The quilt has strength and beauty, and so did our brother. Dick made a difference in our lives, and there was joy in recognizing that difference in a special way. There was joy in being with my family to express together our love and our anguish, and there was a paradoxical joy in being part of the suffering of the larger human family. So, we celebrated our own faith, hope, love and endurance in the midst of sadness and mystery.

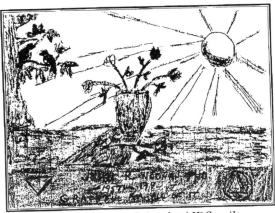

Dick's own sketch for the AIDS quilt

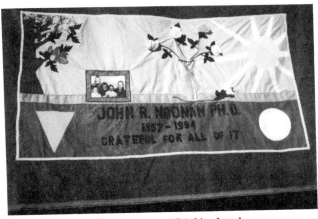

Our implementation of Dick's sketch

Books by Canticle Press
Mail Order Form

Two Children Who Knew Jesus $6.95
by Eileen Lomasney, CSJ
Light From Another Room $10.00
by Eileen Lomasney, CSJ
Jiggle Your Heart and Tickle Your Soul $10.00
(The Uses of Joy and Laughter in Attaining Health and Happiness)
by Anne Bryan Smollin, CSJ
Polish Your Soul and Spruce Up Your Heart $10.00
(How to Like What You See in the Mirror)
by Anne Bryan Smollin, CSJ
The Singing Bird Will Come: An AIDS Journal $10.95
by John R. Noonan, Ph.D., edited by Mary Rose Noonan, CSJ

Please send the following books:

_____

_____

_____

Name: _____

Address: _____

City: _____State:_____Zip:_____

Phone: _____

Shipping: Please add **$4.00** to your order for shipping and handling of 1-3 books, **$5.00** for 4-6 books, **$6.00** for 7-10 books. For bulk-order discounts, call (518) 783-3604.

Sales Tax: Please add sales tax for books shipped to NYS residences or supply tax-exempt number. New York State law requires **8%** sales tax on shipping and handling as well as on merchandise.

Please make checks payable to **Canticle Press, Inc.** and mail to:
Canticle Press, Inc.
385 Watervliet-Shaker Road
Latham, New York 12110-4799